PSYCHOSOCIAL ASPECTS
OF DISABILITY

PSYCHOSOCIAL ASPECTS
OF
DISABILITY

By

GEORGE HENDERSON, Ph.D.

Department of Human Relations
University of Oklahoma
Norman, Oklahoma

and

WILLIE V. BRYAN, Ed.D.

Educational Services
University of Oklahoma
Health Sciences Center
Oklahoma City, Oklahoma

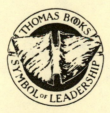

CHARLES C THOMAS • PUBLISHER
Springfield • Illinois • U.S.A.

1984

Published and Distributed Throughout the World by

CHARLES C THOMAS • PUBLISHER
2600 South First Street
Springfield, Illinois 62717

© *1984 by* CHARLES C THOMAS • PUBLISHER

ISBN 0-398-05006-6

Library of Congress Catalog Card Number: 84-2528

With THOMAS BOOKS *careful attention is given to all details of manufacturing and
design. It is the Publisher's desire to present books that are satisfactory as to their physical
qualities and artistic possibilities and appropriate for their particular use.* THOMAS
BOOKS *will be true to those laws of quality that assure a good name and good will.*

Printed in the United States of America
SC-R-3

Library of Congress Cataloging in Publication Data

Henderson, George, 1932–
  Psychosocial aspects of disability.

  Bibliography: p.
  Includes index.
    1. Physically handicapped—Psychology.   2. Physically
handicapped—Rehabilitation—Social aspects.   3. Physically
handicapped—Public opinion.   I. Bryan, Willie V.
II. Title.
RD798.H46   1984   362.4'01'9   84-2528
ISBN 0-398-05006-6

To
Barbara and Donnita

PREFACE

More than thirty million people in the United States have chronic disabilities. These disabilities range from mild to severe, and the largest number of them are found in nine categories: (1) arthritis and rheumatism, (2) heart conditions, (3) hypertension, (4) impaired back and spine, (5) impaired lower extremities, (6) visual impairment, (7) hearing impairment, (8) diabetes, and (9) asthma. The majority of people who have these conditions are not severely disabled, nor are they learning impaired. Yet, they are often identified with those who *do* have severe disabilities. We will discuss both groups, but our major emphasis will be on people who have mild disabilities.

Americans are culturally conditioned to think of persons who have disabilities as being abnormal. This is true even though at least one-fourth of all families have a member with a disability. Even if the incidence of disability were not so great, however, we would be opposed to negative labeling. Our Christian medical ethics decree that all people shall be kept alive whenever possible. However, the Protestant work ethic, which is an integral part of our lives, decrees that the highest level of worker performance is the norm for all workers—persons with and without disabilities. This same work ethic decrees that failure to work when legally able to do so is a sign of inadequacy. Thus, persons with disabilities frequently are kept alive, denied equal opportunity to work, and made to feel guilty for not being optimally productive workers. By any standards of fair play, this is an abominable position.

More often than not, people with physical disabilities are occupationally rather than physically handicapped. Their handicap is primarily attributable to cultural restraints rather than their physical limitations. In every other aspect except physical disability, they are normal people. With the proper rehabilitation, they can become employable. These are the people to whom we devote a major portion of our book, describing their problems and prescribing remedies. Our major focus is on not physical disabilities *per se* but the varying responses to them. If given the chance, we believe, most people can become integral members of their communities. Our focus is on a humanistic approach to helping.

Humanistic approaches to helping can best be understood within the context of humanistic psychology. At its 1963 organizational meeting, the American Association for Humanistic Psychology defined *humanistic psychology* as

> the third main branch of the general field of psychology...and as such...primarily concerned with those human capacities and potentialities that have little or no systematic place, either in positivist or behaviorist theory or in classical psychoanalytic theory, e.g., love, creativity, self, growth, organism, basic need gratification, higher values, being, becoming, spontaneity, play, humor, affection, naturalness, warmth, ego-transcendence, objectivity, autonomy, responsibility, meaning, fair-play, transcendental experience, psychological health, and related concepts.*

From this definition, it is apparent that humanistic psychology seeks to identify and elevate human interests, values, and dignity. Through the integration of related disciplines such as sociology, psychiatry, and education, helpers with a humanistic orientation strive to understand and improve human relations by employing methods that are unswervingly anthropocentric. This model is used in this book.

Depending on the point of view that is emphasized, this approach has been called *humanistic, existential, perceptual, transactional,* and *proactive.* Although the persons involved in humanistic helping do not speak with a single voice, nor do they all specialize in the same content areas, they are united by and committed to the common goal of humanizing society. A major impetus lending dynamic force to the creation of this movement was the prevailing psychological conception of humans as having little freedom of choice or uniqueness among members of the animal species. Also,

---

*From A. J. Satich, Articles of Association, American Association for Humanistic Psychology. Palo Alto, CA, 1963, p. 1.

tradition psychology was characterized as having a dwindling interest in consciousness and a preoccupation with conditioned response and other physiological processes.

The humanistic psychology movement was created to introduce a fresh perspective to psychology rather than formulating a new psychology. The past decade has witnessed a restoration of the whole-person concept to helping. James Bugental (1964), who served as the first president of the American Association for Humanistic Psychology, listed four basic assumptions of humanistic psychology:

- Man, as man, supersedes the sum of his parts.
- Man has his being in a human context.
- Man has choice.
- Man is intentional[*]

These assumptions are adopted and incorporated into our book.

An overview of socioeconomic and psychological factors related to disabilities is presented. By design, we move from general concepts to practical how-to suggestions. Topics discussed briefly in the first few chapters are treated again, but in greater detail, in later chapters. This approach should not be thought of as repetition; rather, it is a way of expanding on relevant issues and topics. Our approach is in harmony with the psychological principle that growth and learning are continuous.

To date, no book focusing on this topic is complete. We did not intend this one to be, either. Rather, we have attempted to build a foundation upon which can be built useful knowledge and helpful behaviors that will improve the quality of life for people with disabilities. Within this framework, we have utilized materials from several excellent social and behavioral sciences books, articles, and papers. By emphasizing practical approaches to helping, we have tried to write a book that will be a reference for all persons concerned about the plight of people with disabilities.

No curriculum or in-service training program is complete without materials that focus on the dynamics of helping, being helpers, and being helped. This, then, is a book for human services person-

---

[*]J. F. T. Bugental. The third force in psychology. *J Human Psychol, 4:* 9, 1964.

nel as well as people with disabilities and their parents, relatives, and friends. We do not view *Psychosocial Aspects of Disability* as competing with the more traditional, heavily research-oriented books. Rather, it has been written to complement and supplement them.

We are grateful to the many persons whose ideas and concepts we cite in the pages that follow. It is gratifying to see the growing concern for improving the quality of life for people with disabilities. Our special thanks go to Professor Clayton Morgan, Coordinator of the Counselor Rehabilitation Training Program at Oklahoma State University, Bernard Posner, Executive Director of the President's Committee on Employment of the Handicapped, and Larry Bishop, Legislative Liaison, Oklahoma Office of Handicapped Concerns, for their thoughtful critiques and suggestions.

This book is our way of saying, "Enough! Let us reach out and help our neighbors with disabilities and help them to help themselves." This is not much to ask, but it will be everything to refuse.

CONTENTS

PSYCHOSOCIAL ASPECTS
OF DISABILITY

Chapter 1

MYTHS AND TREATMENT

In the 1880s, P. T. Barnum earned a small fortune by exhibiting what society had chosen to label *freaks*. In what he called The Greatest Show on Earth, "normal" performers did spectacular things, but it was the freaks who drew the crowds. Throughout history, people without disabilities have had a paradoxical repulsion-attraction for those with disabilities. Faried Haj (1970) cautioned that crude negative attitudes toward the disabled, once deeply rooted in the superstitions and mythologies of the ancestors of modern man, have evolved into present-day sophisticated bigotry.

The collective attempt of the human race to understand its own existence is a classical study in frustration. This notwithstanding, human beings continually do try to understand disability by extracting its significance in the past and, based on that, imposing upon the present a human pecking order that is shaped by their physical health expectations of the future. Despite the time gaps that separate the past, present, and future, the lives of people who have disabilities testify to mind-boggling cruelty over prolonged periods of time. Such inhumanity prompted artist-philosopher Samuel Beckett (1965) to observe, "Yesterday is not a milestone that has been passed but a daystone on the beaten track of the years, and irremediably a part of us, within us, heavy and dangerous" (p. 3).

People's attempts to define and relate practically to the disabilities of themselves and others are understandably difficult. More than likely, confrontations with people who are physically different arouse complex emotions. Most people are saddened by accidents that impair once-healthy individuals and puzzled by infants with disabilities who have "normal" parents. They are frightened by diseases that immobilize the body but leave the mind active and

3

terrified when they realize how vulnerable the human body is to injury. Physical disabilities seem to have a complexity beyond man's powers of total comprehension or cure.

> It is possible that if we examine our own feelings regarding limitations such as blindness, deafness, cerebral palsy, epilepsy, crippling diseases, and others, we will find that we still believe, as did our ancestors, that their basic causes lie in the transgressions of parents, their lack of good judgment, or the punishment for their sins. We are certain that these conditions must be inherited and even contagious. For those who believe these things, a reaction and response to disability of revulsion, avoidance and fear is understandable. Comprehensible, too, then is our insistence that the different be segregated in order that "decent society" may be protected from them. [Buscaglia, 1975, p. 172]

ANCIENT BELIEFS AND TREATMENT

Based in part on the need to survive, primitive societies were intolerant of the physically weak. The individual did not count; the welfare of the group came before all other needs (Apton, 1959). Thus, anyone who was not physically strong enough to contribute to meeting group needs was expendable. This was certainly a period of the survival of the fittest. In primitive societies, persons with disabilities were economic, military, and social liabilities that few groups could afford or, at least, thought they could afford (Hinshaw, 1948).

EVIL SPIRITS. Whenever people must eke their existence from the environment using speed, crude tools, and physical prowess, those who have disabilities become an endangered group. Most primitive people tried to get rid of sick and deformed individuals who did not contribute to the survival of the group by avoiding evil spirits thought to reside in the bodies of such individuals. Long before organized religions, modern man's ancestors were guided by superstitions and folklore.

The religious beliefs and practices of primitive societies were, for the most part, animistic and reflected preoccupation with *mana*, a term adopted by anthropologists. Mana encapsulates the primitive belief in a powerful, invisible, all-pervading force at work in the universe, which could cripple and kill at will. Thus, mental illnesses and physical afflictions were generally viewed as the work of evil mana, or spirits. If, after considerable coaxing, the spirits did not leave a possessed body, this was believed to be indisputable evidence that the individual was being punished. In order to prevent contamination, people possessed with evil spirits were to be either avoided or killed.

There was no single regional or ethnic treatment of people with disabilities. Buscaglia (1975) wrote that the Masai Indians murdered such individuals. The Chagga of East Africa believed they had special powers and used them to ward off evil spirits; the Jukum of Sudan said that people with disabilities were the work of evil spirits. The Sem Ang of Malaysia used men with disabilities, whom they considered to be "wise men," for settling tribal disputes, while the Balinese made them taboo. The Hebrews defined them as sinners; the Nordics called them gods.

ABANDONMENT AND DEATH. Historical records reveal that as civilization replaced primitivism, a few other ways to deal with people with disabilities did evolve. They were accepted and treated well in a few ancient societies. In France during the Middle Ages, the blind occupied a place of privilege. Progressive physicians in the Mediterranean region and Asia demanded that people with physical disabilities be treated in a humane manner. However, the people in most countries still treated persons with disabilities much as their ancestors had. Whatever humane enlightenment was occurring in these countries, little of it was extended to the treatment of people with disabilities.

In the Far East, infants with disabilities were abandoned to die in the wilderness. In India, they were drowned in the Ganges River. Roman fathers ritualistically displayed children who had disabilities and, after at least five persons concurred that the children would be of no benefit to society, killed them. In later times, Roman fathers were authorized to make this decision without consultation. Small baskets sold in markets were used as death boats so that children with disabilities could be set sail on the Tiber River. Infants of Sparta suffered a similar fate. If, after being examined by a committee of elders, certain infants were judged as incapable of contributing to society, they were killed. Infanticide was a popular method used by the nobility to eliminate persons whose disabilities might weaken their family's bloodlines. In Athens, special clay pots were used as depositories for abandoned infants.

Many of the children with disabilities who were spared such fatal parental judgment roamed the villages and countrysides as gypsies and beggars. Some of them were taken in by other families and subjected to conditions of slavery; others were forced into prostitution. Although a few persons with disabilities were treated well, they were not immune from abandonment, savage beatings, or death as punishment for being different. In somewhat of a macabre turnabout, some societies considered it honorable for children to kill, cook and eat, or bury alive their aged parents or other relatives who were considered unfit for work or war (Koestler, 1976).

Shifts in Beliefs and Treatment

The rise of humanism, empiricism, and secularism during the Renaissance ushered in more tolerant attitudes and improved treatment of people with disabilities (Rubin and Roessler, 1978). For example, the Elizabethan English Poor Laws, enacted between 1597 and 1601, served as the legal foundation upon which the poor and disabled were protected from many of the harsh and degrading treatments of earlier times. In addition, these laws mandated financial support for persons who were involuntarily unemployed, including individuals with disabilities.

This change of attitude is best seen in the treatment of the deaf. Deaf children were taught to write in the early part of the fifteenth century. Such efforts gradually led to a shift in the perception of people with disabilities, from defining them as totally worthless to believing that they were capable of learning and therefore could become marginally productive members of society. This shift was significant in human relations. Building on such success in the fifteenth century, numerous deaf people in the sixteenth century not only were taught to write but also were taught to read, speak, and understand arithmetic.

Despite this progress, in early American history, severe limitations in the medical knowledge and resources available to people with disabilities resulted in a lack of treatment in their homes or private charity houses. The quality of medical care in the colonies precluded significant rehabilitation. Although the state of the art of medicine was a considerable improvement over primitive methods such as casting spells, there was still little scientific knowledge about germs, and almost nothing was known about the causes of some disabilities. Colonial physicians, often self-trained, usually tried to rid the body of diseases such as typhoid fever and influenza by inducing nausea. Bleeding was another widespread, "advanced" method of medical treatment, used to cleanse the blood of infections.

Fortunately, medical knowledge and, therefore, treatment of patients began to improve in the nineteenth century. Medical schools started requiring their students to study in laboratories and prove their competency by passing examinations. As medical personnel learned more about the causes of disabling conditions, they began to demand better facilities to treat people with disabilities. In India there were many hospitals that were fully equipped for treating people who had disabilities. A hospital in Baghdad offered the most modern treatment of the period. The Egyptians and Greeks also began to build hospitals and convalescent centers to care for people with disabilities. One hospital in Cairo provided free treatment, and, upon discharge, patients were given money to sustain them until they could secure work.

However, these were exceptional cases. Although some nineteenth-century physicians advocated humane treatment of patients with disabilities, the majority of them contributed to the negative attitudes and even administered inhumane treatment themselves. Lacking scientific methods to determine the origin of diseases, early physicians did little to explode the myth that physiologic disorders were the result of evil spirits. Consequently, common "cures" continued to include bleeding, potions, and ostracism.

Before the Civil War, three hospitals in New York and Philadelphia provided care for people with disabilities. In 1837, the first sheltered workshop for people with disabilities was established. The Perkins Institute of Boston was set up to train blind people so that they could work in the community. Toward the end of the nineteenth century, a group of Cleveland, Ohio women, known as the Sunbeam Circle, made and sold handiwork and used the profits to help the crippled children of Cleveland. A few years later, the Cleveland Rehabilitation Center became a forerunner of modern rehabilitation centers. Although the Center's initial efforts focused on helping children with disabilities, it later expanded to include adults.

Other well-known private organizations began during this period. The Salvation Army, for example, began in England in 1878 and expanded to the United States in 1880. In 1902, the Goodwill Industries was organized in this country by Edgar J. Helms, a Methodist minister. Primarily individual religious groups initiated major efforts to get persons with disabilities into the mainstream of society. The first totally American, state-supported institution designed to aid the poor was established in 1897—the Minnesota State Hospital for Indigent and Dependent Children. Although it was not set up exclusively for patients with disabilities, this hospital treated a substantial number of them because private care was unaffordable.

Biblical and Other Literature

Many of the ancient myths and stereotypes of people with disabilities still exist. Although few persons currently subscribe to abandoning or killing people with disabilities, many do associate disabilities with sin and the Devil. They either consciously or subconsciously think that *disability* is a synonym of *bad.* More often than not, *able-bodied* is associated with *good,* i.e. Christ and the angels, cleanliness, and virtue. None of the great artists ever created images of angels with disabilities. Conversely, persons with disabilities have been associated through the ages with all that is bad. A review of literature reveals that at various times physical disabilities have stood for dirt, sin, and evil.

Metaphoric usages of disabled as evil and able-bodied as goodness appear abundantly throughout the Bible. They are also ingrained in the writings of ancient and contemporary literature and, indeed, are symbolically woven into almost every reference to health. Positive images of nondisabled and negative images of disabled have been etched deep in the minds of most people throughout history, and many able-bodied persons have nourished these images in order to maintain their own sense of self-esteem.

Much like the English child in an Edwin Blake poem, the able-bodied perceive themselves as angels, while persons with disabilities can only yearn for wholeness through their character or deeds, hoping to become like the able-bodied so that they will at last be accepted as worthy beings. This socially perverse arrangement is communicated through social status, peer relationships, education, and job opportunities. This concept is carefully and religiously injected into children through school texts, television programs, and catechism. Nancy Weinberg and Carol Sebian (1980) offered the following excellent overview of passages from the Bible that support negative views of people with physical disabilities:

> Throughout the Bible the notion recurs that disease and physical disabilities are punishments sent by God for sins or immoral behavior. God revealed His law through the writings of prophets and disciples. Those who obeyed God's law thrived in good health; those who transgressed against His commandments were severely punished. In the Old Testament, Deut. 27:27, God admonished people to obey all His commandments or He would inflict them with blindness. The New Testament restates the same sentiment that physical illness and disability are punishments for some religious transgression. In John 5:14, Jesus upon healing a man said, "See, you are well? Sin no more, that nothing more befall you." In Matthew 9:2, Jesus said to a man with palsy, "My son, your sins are forgiven." These teachings imply that the sick and disabled deserve to suffer as a punishment for having sinned. Not only can the individual sinner be punished, but divine retribution can also be directed toward the innocent offspring of a sinner. This is demonstrated in an incident from the Book of Samuel: David said to Nathan, "I have sinned against the Lord," and Nathan said to David, "The Lord also has put away your sin; you shall not die. Nevertheless, because by this deed you have utterly scorned the Lord, the child that is born to you shall die." And the Lord struck the child that Ureah's wife bore to David, and it became sick and on the seventh day the child was dead. [P. 273]

Other forms of literature have also contributed to the negative image of persons with disabilities. For example, the Talmud and other Hebrew commentaries refer to the blind as the "living dead." A Talmudic commandment urges those who meet a blind person to say the same prayer as would be said upon the death of a close relative. The belief that disability is synonymous with worthlessness, shame, and pity is displayed poetically in lines of numerous writings, including John Milton's (1671) poem "Samson Agonistes":

> Now blind-disheartn'd sham'd
> dishonor's quell'd
> To what can I be useful, wherein
> serve my nation, and the work from
> Heav'n impos'd
> But to sit idle on the household hearth
> A burdenous drone; to visetonts a gaze,
> or pitied object.

In *Lady Chatterley's Lover,* D. H. Lawrence (1930) perpetuated the idea of disability as equivalent to uselessness. In it, Sir Clifford, after being injured in war, becomes impotent and therefore is depicted as not being a "whole" man. (*See* Chapter 4 of this volume for other illustrations of literary treatment of the disabled.)

Myths and stereotypes do not necessarily depict persons with disabilities negatively. Unfounded positive images are also part of the mystique of people with disabilities. For example, it is commonly believed that nature automatically compensates blind individuals by sharpening their other senses. Helen Keller was assured by her friends that blind people can identify colors by touch. Many other positive traits are attributed to persons with disabilities solely on the basis of this "automatic compensation" myth. Some of the more desirable mythical traits are cheerfulness, patience, and extraordinary musical skills. Although these myths positively reflect persons with disabilities, they are nevertheless as inaccurate and distorted as the negative myths. The deaf have no better eyesight than the nondeaf; they simply learn to pay attention to more things. The blind have no better hearing than the sighted; they learn to use their ears more efficiently.

Many persons have expressed difficulty accepting as sincere the statements of respondents who publicly proclaim their pride in having a disability because such persons often discover that pride alone cannot overcome disability barriers. Not even rewriting the literature can do that. The conflicts that result from disability do not lead to a single response: Some individuals withdraw; others clown; many become aggressive or highly suspicious of people without disabilities; and still others assume proud mannerisms. Those who are able to accept the label *disabled* do not find utopia; an invisible veil prevents them from being treated like first-class citizens.

LEGISLATIVE ACTION

In 1917, Congress passed the Smith-Hughes Act, a landmark education act that set the precedent for subsequent federal funding of educational programs, not only for people with disabilities but also for other people (Cull and Hardy, 1973). In addition, it called for a Board of Vocational Education to spearhead the drive for vocational education. This board was to become the foundation for vocational rehabilitation in the United States. The first Board of Vocational Education was funded in 1918 under the Soldier Rehabilitation Act to operate a program of vocational rehabilitation for World War I veterans. Better known as the Smith-Sears Veterans' Rehabilitation Act of 1918, it provided the following general purview for federal vocational rehabilitation services: "An act to provide for the vocational rehabilitation and return to employment of disabled persons discharged from the military or naval forces of the United States and for other purposes."

After this seed had been planted, state and federal vocational rehabilitation programs developed. However, before these programs evolved to their present status, they progressed through several stages.

SMITH-FESS ACT (1920). President Woodrow Wilson's signature on PL-236 (the Smith-Fess Act) in 1920 made public rehabilitation programs a long-awaited reality. This act established federal and state rehabilitation programs and provided for an equal sharing of expenditures for them. The act was not without limitations, however. Funds were provided only for vocational guidance, training, occupational adjustment, prostheses, and placement services. In short, rehabilitation services for persons with physical disabilities were to be vocational in nature; physical restoration and sociopsychologic services were excluded.

Actually, the Smith-Fess Act was an extension of earlier vocational education legislation. It added the provision making rehabilitation services available to people with physical disabilities. Also, this was temporary legislation and remained operative only by additional legislation. In 1924, federal legislation was passed that extended the life of state and federal vocational rehabilitation programs for an additional six years. It was not until the 1935 Federal Social Security Act that state and federal vocational rehabilitation programs became permanent. The long and tedious battle to institutionalize vocational rehabilitation for the disabled was finally won.

BARDEN-LaFOLLETTE ACT (1943). More commonly known as the Vocational Rehabilitation Act of 1943, the Barden-LaFollette Act strengthened vocational rehabilitation programs by providing physical restoration services to people with disabilities. In addition, it extended vocational rehabilitation services to the mentally handicapped and the mentally ill. In 1954 this act was again amended, and the following significant changes made:

1. More funds and additional program options were provided to state agencies.
2. Federally funded research programs were established.
3. Training funds were added for physicians, nurses, rehabilitation counselors, physical therapists, occupational therapists, social workers, psychologists, and other specialists in the field of rehabilitation.

VOCATIONAL REHABILITATION ACT AMENDMENTS (1965). These amendments further strengthened vocational rehabilitation programs by (1) providing monies to states for innovative projects that developed new methods of providing services and otherwise serving persons with severe disabilities; (2) creating a broader base of services to persons with disabilities, including individuals with socially handicapping conditions; and (3) eliminating economic need as a requisite for rehabilitation services. Slowly, the related pieces to comprehensive care were coming together to form a meaningful whole.

REHABILITATION ACT OF 1973. PL-112 of the Ninety-third Congress replaced the Vocational Rehabilitation Act as amended in 1968 with this new act, which maintained the major provisions of the 1968 amended act and added the provision that before receiving funds a state must conduct a thorough study to determine the needs of its handicapped citizens. Other significant provisions of the act were the inclusion in Title V of Sections 501, 502, 503, and 504.

Section 501. This section established the Interagency Committee on Handicapped Employees. The Committee consists of federal agency heads, who have the responsibility to review annually the adequacy of federal hiring, placement, and job advancement of persons with disabilities. Based on each review, the Committee can recommend further legislation and administrative changes.

Section 502. This section established the Architectural and Transportation Barriers Compliance Board, which has the responsibility of monitoring the construction of new federal buildings and the remodeling of old ones to ensure that they are accessible to persons with physical disabilities. Existing federal buildings that are not being remodeled do not have to be made accessible.

Section 503. The words *affirmative action* were introduced into the vocabulary of rehabilitation in Section 503, which requires that every employer doing business with the federal government under a contract for more than $2,500 take affirmative action in hiring persons with disabilities. Throughout the various stages of employment (recruiting, hiring, upgrading, transferring, advertising for recruitment, establishing rates of pay, and selecting persons for apprenticeships), affirmative action must be taken.

Section 504. If the law contained within Section 504 were followed to the letter, at least 80 percent of the employment problems of persons with physical disabilities would vanish. This section calls for nondiscrimination in employment. Every United States institution that receives federal financial assistance must take steps to ensure that people with disabilities are not discriminated against in employment.

It is important to note that the enactment of Sections 503 and 504 began a major change in America's national commitment to citizens with disabilities. In the 1980s, these laws are more symbolic than concrete. They codify the concept that all people have the right to reach their full potential.

The Rehabilitation Act of 1973 was amended in 1974 and 1978. The 1974 amendments significantly strengthened programs for the blind that were first authorized in 1936 by the Randolph-

Shepard Act. (This act had authorized states to license qualified blind persons to operate vending stands in federal buildings.) In addition to providing increased funding to states, some provisions of the amendments to the Rehabilitation Act of 1973 focused on employment opportunities and independent living for people with disabilities. Specifically, the provisions provided for (1) community service employment pilot programs; (2) projects with industry and business to accelerate the training and employment of persons with disabilities; (3) grants and contracts with individuals with disabilities to start or operate business enterprises; (4) loans from the Small Business Administration to persons with disabilities when other financial assistance is not available; (5) funds for comprehensive services for independent living for individuals with severe disabilities; and (6) grants to states for the establishment and operation of independent living centers.

PEOPLE WITH DISABILITIES IN THE WORLD OF WORK

Despite the momentous efforts of dedicated individuals and private and public organizations to treat people with disabilities with dignity rather than as clowns, freaks, and objects of pity, negative myths and stereotypes persist. Persons with disabilities are often regarded as useless or less adequate than those without disabilities. Such perceptions impede efforts to move people with disabilities into the mainstream of local, state, and national activities.

Significant changes have occurred in the concept of *work* since prehistoric days, when people had to work only enough to meet very basic needs for food, clothing, and shelter. As time passed and human needs became more symbolic, work and work-related activities began to take on meanings that went beyond basic survival. The earliest recorded ideas about work referred to it as a curse, a punishment, an activity not included as part of the good life, and at best a necessary evil—needed to sustain life (Lofquist and Dawis, 1969). People of high status did not work. Only slaves, indentured servants, and peasants worked. The masters or ruling classes did not work; they were preoccupied with intellectual contemplation that could not be sustained through physical labor. In summary, work was considered necessary, but only insofar as to sustain the individual and the group to which he or she belonged.

The Protestant Work Ethic

As Christianity spread, the meaning of *work* began to change. Martin Luther subscribed to the principle that work is a form of redemption. The religious decree was that all people who are able to work *should* work, including affluent intellectuals and ascetics. Thus, whether an individual's economic position was high or low, he or she was expected to work in order to serve God. According to Luther, the best way to serve God was by performing work more perfectly. The philosophies of John Calvin and Luther were very similar in regard to work, which they both thought curbed the evil in people. Max Weber (1930) stated that the belief that work was the highest means of asceticism and the strongest proof of religious faith had the greatest influence in shaping capitalism. Work became the religious spirit of capitalism and had at least three basic meanings for preindustrial people: (1) It was hard, necessary and burdensome; (2) it was a means to religious fulfillment; and (3) it was good because it was a creative act.

Noted scholars in the field of occupation and career development (e.g. Roe, 1956; Super, 1968; Deutscher, 1971) observed that the meaning of *work* changed in the twentieth century. In the 1980s, work is valued as a way to get consumer goods and maintain dignity and self-esteem rather than as verification of religious salvation. In discussing the importance and meaning of work in modern society, C. Esco Obermann (1965) concluded that the most observable contributions by individuals to their society are made through their work or occupations. In technologic cultures, work or occupation more nearly defines a person's importance. Consequently, job success is likely to help satisfy the need for recognition and status. In the 1980s, occupation is one of the most important aspects of an individual's life; it defines his or her place in the community. Generally, social status, technical capabilities, and economic level—all evolve from occupation. What about persons with disabilities, who tend to be unemployed and underemployed?

Self-esteem

In the second century, Galen wrote, "Employment is nature's best physician, an essential to happiness." With the advent of the Industrial Revolution and the beginning of the Age of Automation, humans became concerned with the relevance of work to their search for identity. Although no society still subscribes to the idea of hard work for all, most societies promote the idea that work for the able-bodied is good. A Gallup Poll reported the following comments about public assistance (Wolfbein, 1971):

> If we give people money without working we will be taking away the individual's incentive to work and his ability to pass this incentive on to his children. To do this would be creating a society of parasites—a something for nothing society.

> I don't want my tax money going to someone who is sitting around with his feet up in the air. I feel they should be provided with a job, not charity. This gives a man confidence by letting him earn the money thus making him feel like a man. [P. 164]

The same Gallup Poll asked "Would you favor a guaranteed income?" Fifty-eight percent of the respondents disapproved. However, to the question, "Do you favor providing enough work for everyone?" 82 percent answered in the affirmative, which reflects an American tradition—the belief that work is good and that through work, man is contributing to society.

According to Childs (1971), work is more than a means through which goods and services are purchased; it is a means by which an individual purchases his or her dignity. Through work, identity and social status are achieved. One of the questions almost always asked of strangers in casual conversation is, "What is your job?" The answer to that usually sparks a mental picture that categorizes the individual. Max Deutscher (1971) offered a cogent analysis of the importance of work in the development of self-esteem: Involvement with meaningful work is an adult activity. It helps to establish and maintain adult life. It is not that people work *when* they become adults, but that they work *to become* adults, to nourish the adult personality structure with its capacity for intimacy, relatedness, productivity, and participation in community life. Work provides a much-needed link to reality in nonchild contexts.

Furthermore, it has a fundamental economic reality: Most people have to work in order to provide financial support for themselves and their families. Finally, work has social reality. Through work, people earn a place in their community and develop within themselves a sense of accomplishment. Indeed, work status shapes nonjob actions. What about people who have disabilities?

Humans work to help satisfy the basic needs set forth in Abraham Maslow's (1954) hierarchy of needs, as explained by Ann Roe (1956):

> In our society, there is no single situation which is potentially so capable of giving some satisfaction at all levels of basic needs as is the occupation. With respect to the physiological needs, it is clear that in our culture the usual means for allaying hunger and thirst, and to some extent, sexual needs and the others is through the job, which provides the money that can be exchanged for food and drink. The same is true for the safety needs. The need to be a member of a group and to give and receive love is also one which can be satisfied in part by the occupation. To work with a congenial group, to be an extrinsic part of the function to the group, to be needed and welcomed by the group are important aspects of the satisfactory job.
>
> Perhaps satisfaction of the need for esteem from self and others is most easily seen as a big part of the occupation. In the first place, entering upon an occupation is generally seen in our culture as a symbol of adulthood, and an indication that a young man or woman has reached a stage of some independence and freedom. Having a job in itself carries a measure of esteem. What importance it has is seen most clearly in the devastating effects upon the individual of being out of work.
>
> Occupations as a source of need satisfaction are of extreme importance in our culture. It may be that occupations have become so important in our culture just because so many needs are so well satisfied by them. [Pp. 31–32]

Congress recognized, when it amended the Social Security Act in 1967, that doling out funds to unemployed people who are able to work does very little to bolster their self-esteem. The amendments required parents of dependent children to be involved in job training or work. Every state is legally required to deny welfare payments to any father or mother who is considered able to work or engage in training but who rejects training or work opportunities. Summarizing these ideas, Emanuel Friedman and Robert Havighurst (1954) listed several common meanings of *work:*

1. It is a source of self-respect, a way of achieving recognition or respect from others.
2. It defines a person's identity, his role in society.
3. It provides the opportunity for association with other persons for building friendships.
4. It allows for self-expression and provides the opportunity for creativity and new experiences.
5. It permits people to be of service to others.

Individuals tend to want an occupation that would likely permit them self-expression. The manner in which occupational self-expression is implemented is, to a great extent, determined by external conditions.

Work takes on increased meaning for people who have disabilities (Vash, 1981). Such individuals are viewed as not being capable persons when so much emphasis is put on physical abilities. Indeed, many prospective employers believe that persons who are disabled are less than normal. These employers are likely to recall a negative stereotype of physically disabled people and consequently expect less of workers with disabilities. They also often believe that persons with disabilities should expect less of themselves. Because of this kind of thinking, few people are surprised when a person with a disability reports that he or she cannot get a job.

Getting a Job

Work is a basic ingredient in modern culture; most people organize their lives around their occupations. Grave psychologic disturbances can result when persons with disabilities who are able to work are barred from participating in this most important societal activity. When individuals are unable to find or keep a job because of prejudices about their disabilities, physical disability becomes a handicap. The work capabilities of most persons with physical disabilities have been demonstrated many times. There are several factors more important for the performance of most jobs than physical prowess.

In the early 1960s, the staff of the Vocational Rehabilitation

Division of the Federal Board for Vocational Education studied 6,097 persons with physical disabilities who were employed after being rehabilitated. The investigation confirmed that (1) rehabilitated persons could perform adequately in a wide range of occupations; (2) persons with disabilities, even those with similar diagnoses, differed greatly from each other in many occupational factors; and (3) it is not possible to equate disability and occupational capability (Obermann, 1965). During this same period, Roe (1956) said the following about persons with disabilities and their ability to work:

> Unlike special abilities which may qualify their holder for desirable, unusual jobs, special disabilities are more likely to function as only limited factors. Blindness, deafness, orthopedic disabilities, chronic illness all have very real effects upon occupational selection. Some of these effects, it is true, are the result of inadequate knowledge on the part of everyone, the disabled, the employers and society generally, as to just what performance limitations are the necessary results of certain disabilities, but some of the effects are genuinely inevitable. A man with one arm cannot perform activities which really require two fully functional ones, but he can do many more things with one arm and one prosthetic device than might be imagined. Furthermore, there are a large number of occupations for which a second arm is really unnecessary. [Pp. 64–65]

Through the years, individual and group prejudices based on unfounded myths have caused workers with disabilities to be relegated to dead-end jobs, if any at all. This negative attitude is the greatest hurdle that people with disabilities have to overcome, and it is an extremely high hurdle, built on actual disabilities as well as imagined ones. As long as the Puritan work ethic is attached to mores and behaviors concerning the worth of individuals, it will be through work that persons with disabilities become contributing members of society. Most individuals with disabilities strongly desire to live up to societal standards of being economically productive citizens. However, traditional attitudes toward them do not facilitate this. Even the schools treat them as less capable people. Moreover, of course, persons with disabilities themselves often consider their plight as being inevitable.

Because this nation suffers from a lack of understanding of the wants, needs, and capabilities of people with disabilities, not enough pressure is put on schools to teach them properly and on employers to hire them. In the same vein as the "Sunday Christian," who sins during the week but feels that he has discharged his religious duties by attending church on Sunday, many educators and employers believe that they fulfill their obligations to the disabled by donating money to charity drives. Despite educators' and employers' awareness of the therapeutic value of education and work, it is still difficult to find effective teachers and gainful employment for individuals with disabilities. As the twenty-first century approaches, it is sad that old myths and stereotypes continue to thwart many citizens' quest for dignity and equality. Those who succeed usually do so at a tremendously high personal cost.

Myths hurt people with disabilities who want to work. These myths are discussed in the next few pages because the authors of this book believe that the reluctance of employers to hire workers with disabilities stems primarily from false assumptions that are deeply entrenched. (*See* Nathanson, 1979, for refutation of these assumptions.) Common myths relate to safety, insurance, liability, productivity, attendance, accommodations, and acceptance in the work force.

Safety Myth

Myth: Because workers with disabilities deviate from what employers generally consider normal, i.e. they walk differently, walk with the aid of something, or have a hearing or visual impairment, they are likely to injure themselves or cause other employees to be injured.

Reality: In 1981, a survey conducted by the DuPont Company showed that, with respect to safety, 96 percent of their employees with disabilities rated average or above average, compared with 92 percent for employees who did not have disabilities. Other studies have also indicated that individuals with disabilities are safe employees. A 1978 International Telephone and Telegraph Company (ITT) study of their Corinth, Mississippi plant, where 125 persons with disabilities were part of a 2,000-member work force, showed an all-time safety record of 3,700,000 man-hours worked without lost time that was injury related. At the time of the survey, no worker with a disability had suffered more than a minor on-the-job injury since starting with the company (President's Committee on Employment of the Handicapped, 1982). Other large companies such as IBM, Sears and Roebuck, and ConEd have been leaders in hiring the handicapped. If these companies had not found them to be safe workers, they would not continue to recruit and hire them. Employers' past experience with workers who have disabilities correlates positively with their readiness to hire them (Florian, 1978).

Insurance Myth

Myth: Insurance companies will not let employers hire workers with disabilities. "My insurance company will penalize me if I hire a disabled person. My insurance rates will go up. My workmen's compensation rates will go up."

Reality: Insurance companies do not tell employers whom to hire, nor are employers required to get approval for workmen's compensation insurance before hiring disabled workers (Brantman, 1978). Insurance premiums are based on a company's safety record, not its workers' physiques. As discussed in regard to the safety myth, employees with disabilities are proportionately as safe as, if not safer than, workers who do not have disabilities. Aware of this, the insurance industry does not oppose but actually encourages the employment of individuals with disabilities. Workers' compensation insurance rates are determined by three factors: (1) nature of the business, (2) size of payroll, and, for larger employers, (3) accident experience. In determining workmen's compensation insurance rates, occupations are classified so that the cost of accidents can be assessed proportionately to the accident risks involved. Hazardous occupations have higher workmen's compensation rates than sedentary occupations.

The DuPont Company did not experience an increase in workmen's compensation or health, accident, or other medical insurance costs. A recent survey of 279 companies made by the United States Chamber of Commerce and the National Association of Manufacturers revealed that 90 percent of the respondents reported no change in insurance costs as a result of hiring persons with disabilities (President's Committee on Employment of the Handicapped, 1982).

Liability Myth

Myth: An on-the-job accident that, when added to a worker's prior disability, results in permanent total disability will make the company liable for permanent total disability.

Reality: All fifty states and the District of Columbia now have a Second Injury Fund built into their workers' compensation law. The Second Injury Fund assumes the responsibility of compensation to a person with a physical disability who becomes totally disabled through an industrial accident, allocating to the employer's expense only the single injury sustained at work. Because each state develops its own Second Injury Fund, specific provisions and the way they are applied vary from state to state.

Productivity Myth

Myth: Workers with disabilities are not capable of performing their jobs; therefore, the other employees have to "take up the slack."

Reality: An employer should know what skills are required to accomplish a job; if applicants with disabilities possess the skills, there is no reason they should not be hired. For example, if a job's primary skill requirement is eye-hand coordination and the applicant is in a wheelchair, assuming he or she has good eye-hand coordination, there is no reason he or she should not be hired. Relatedly, if applicants with disabilities do not possess the required skills but are capable of learning them with reasonable training, there is no reason they should not be hired. Conversely, if applicants with disabilities do not possess the needed skills and training is not feasible, they should not be hired.

Job applicants with physical disabilities should fill out the same employment forms, take the same tests, and be given the same interview as other applicants. In short, they should be given an equal opportunity, but if they do not have the aptitude for the job, they should not be hired. They deserve the same, not unequal, breaks. The DuPont study showed that 92 percent of their workers with disabilities were rated average or above average, compared with 91 percent for their workers who did not have disabilities. ITT found that individuals with disabilities were more productive than their co-workers. These results are similar to findings in other studies (Yuker, Campbell, and Block, 1960; Weissman, 1965).

Attendance Myth

Myth: Workers with disabilities are absent from their jobs a great amount of time because of their physical problems.

Reality: If they are job-ready via physical or vocational rehabilitation, persons with disabilities should have no more absences than other persons. There may be a few exceptions, such as persons with arthritic conditions or allergies, who are affected by climatic changes. ITT discovered that the workers with disabilities in their Corinth plant had fewer absences than their nondisabled co-workers: Eighty-five percent of the workers with disabilities were average or above average in attendance. Persons with disabilities are keenly aware of the difficulty of securing employment; therefore, once they obtain jobs, most of them will not risk losing them by faking illnesses.

Accommodations Myth

Myth: Most job sites would have to be specially redesigned to suit persons with disabilities. "Our company will have to spend a fortune to accommodate disabled workers. They need a lot of special equipment."

Reality: The expenditures that most companies must make to accommodate workers with disabilities are not exorbitant. Once experts evaluate their needs, most organizations are pleasantly surprised at the results. For example, engineers at Kaiser Aluminum estimated it would cost $160,000 to bring their California corporate headquarters into compliance, but a consulting firm reviewed the facilities and concluded that it could be done for less than $8,000 (Koestler, 1980). ITT spent $22,750 at its Corinth plant to make it accessible to individuals with disabilities, and most of that amount ($22,000) was for an elevator. When modifying a corporate headquarters building to aid employees with disabilities, the Rehabilitation Institute of Chicago reduced an outside contractor's estimate for necessary alterations from $96,000 to $5,000. The saving was accomplished by making selective modifications rather than wholesale changes and by doing the work in house.

Sears and Roebuck made structural changes at its executive headquarters to accommodate persons with disabilities for a very modest cost—$300 for cassette tape recorders for six blind telephone salespeople; $800 to lower desks, widen doors, and install restroom grab-bars for catalog order-takers who use wheelchairs; between $300 and $600 for similar accommodations for service technicians in wheelchairs; and $3,800 for a reading machine for the blind and instruction in its use (President's Committee on Employment of the Handicapped, 1982).

Acceptance Myth

Myth: Employees who do not have disabilities will not accept individuals with disabilities. The special accommodations (e.g. parking spaces, wheelchair ramps, and elevators) will be resented.

Reality: The DuPont survey did not find that special accommodations resulted in much resentment of workers with disabilities. Once able-bodied persons work with individuals with disabilities and discover that they are capable of doing their jobs, acceptance or rejection occurs for reasons other than physical disabilities.

SUMMARY

The importance of myths and stereotypes should not be minimized. People with physical disabilities gain much of their inferiority from initially false myths and stereotypes. When employers unequivocally state that individuals with disabilities are poor employees and then either deny them jobs or relegate them to low-paying, dead-end jobs, many of these individuals in fact begin to exhibit inferiority complexes. Vash (1981) concluded:

> Most of us have three types of goals. We want to *get* specific materialistic rewards, such as homes, cars, adult play toys, and so forth. We also want to *do* identified activities, either for the pleasure of the process, the outcomes or both. And we want to *be* a certain way, viewed by ourselves or others as good or honest or tough or whatever characteristics are deemed desirable. Disabled workers have little chance of reaching these goals through their work, or at all, if they are relegated to traditional or conveniently available jobs. [P. 106]

Moreover, if persons with disabilities become a contrast to those without disabilities, then poverty-stricken persons with disabilities become an enigma to all people. In recent years, people with physical disabilities have become a topic for public conferences, frequent subjects for research, and prime recipients of architectural innovations. Each year, they seem to become more infamous and less financially secure (Burdette and Frohlich, 1977). It is not the American dream that is repulsive to unemployed and underemployed people with disabilities but their inability to achieve it. Until this situation changes, many of them are likely to be disgruntled citizens.

DEFINITIONS

The words *disability* and *handicap* are most often used interchangeably. Definitions of words and the way in which they are used often create problems, such as the projection of undesirable images of people. Wright (1960) warned against using shortcuts to describe persons with disabilities: "It is precisely the perception of a person with a physical disability as a physically disabled person that has reduced all his life to the disability aspects of his physique. The shortcut distorts and undermines" (p. 8). She concluded her remarks by pointing out that the use of shortcuts is a major factor in the derogatory connotations of *disabled* and *handicapped.*

Even so, unless they are professionals in a medical field or in some other helping profession, most people do not make a distinction between *disability* and *handicap.* In fact, professional helpers in the field of rehabilitation contributed to the confusion during the many years they used the words *handicapped persons* to identify people they now call *disabled.* Wright argued that using these terms is a shortcut and *individuals with disabilities* and *individuals with handicaps* should be used instead. Is this much ado about nothing? The authors do not think it is.

DISABILITY. Wright (1960) defined a *disability* as "a condition of impairment, physical or mental, having an objective aspect that can usually be described by a physician" (p. 9). James Bitter (1979) added to the definition by pointing out that the physical or mental condition limits a person's activities or functioning. Jeffrey Koshel and Carl Granger (1978) cautioned against the use of unidimensional definitions of *disability:*

Use of the term disabled should assume interaction between the individual and the environment. However, in common usage the word disability is frequently equated with separate and specific physical or mental impairments, or both, thus omitting the contributory effects of the environment. When impairments are viewed as sufficient cause for disability, then the unfortunate use of diagnostic labels as shortcut proxies for disability can lead to a pessimistic outlook regarding the rehabilitative potential of individuals. [P. 102]

HANDICAP. The dictionary defines a *handicap* as a deficiency, especially an anatomical, physiological, or mental deficiency that prevents or restricts normal achievement. Wright added to this definition by stating that a handicap is "the cumulative result of the obstacles which disability interposes between the individual and his maximum function level" (p. 9).

The term *handicapped* should be used only when specific life processes or social activities are adversely affected. That is, an individual can be handicapped in certain aspects of functioning and, at the same time, be fully functional in many others. In most textbooks, Franklin Delano Roosevelt and Helen Keller are used to illustrate this point. There are countless less well known persons whose lives also attest to the relativity of handicaps.

IMPAIRMENT. The definition of *impairment* depends on the functions that are being emphasized. For example, the definitions most commonly used in vocational rehabilitation state that an individual with an impairment is someone who has a physical or mental condition that constitutes or results in hindering employment. Other social institutions define *impairment* in relation to functions that are important to their organizational focus. Succinctly, an impairment is any condition that prevents individuals from adequately performing particular functions that are important to them.

If people have impairments or disorders that are severe enough to constitute a disability or a dysfunctional condition, then it can be said they are handicapped to the degree their social role performance is adversely affected. Even when impairment is constant rather than intermittent, it is possible that an individual may be socially dysfunctional only in a limited way. In short, one cannot know the effects of an impairment without knowing the person with the impairment.

Putting It Together

Although all people with physical disabilities are not handicapped, there is the tendency for others to think of them as being handicapped and for them to think of themselves as being handicapped. Generally, people do not consider children to be handicapped because their physical or mental abilities are less than those of their parents. However, they frequently consider them handicapped if their physical or mental abilities are less than those of their peers. Somewhere in their minds is a nebulous but important concept of the "normal" person, who is able-bodied and visually attractive. To be different is to be set apart, to be abnormal.

"Being different" can include confinement to a wheelchair, slurred speech, impaired vision or hearing, a limp, or a missing part of the body. Interestingly, these differences are comparable to those of ethnic minorities, who may be different because of skin color, language, hair texture, physical features, and religious beliefs.

Individuals who accept definitions of themselves as abnormal usually try to minimize contact with "normal" people or hide their deviance to avoid intruding unnecessarily into social relationships (McDaniel, 1970). Indeed, it is expected by most people that persons with disabilities will know and stay in their place away from their rejectors. As a friend counseled a disabled person: "You're a blind man, now, you'll be expected to act like one. People will be firmly convinced that you consider yourself a tragedy. They'll be disconcerted and even shocked to discover that you don't" (Wright, 1960, p. 15).

Disabilities are deficiencies, and, unfortunately, other persons look down on persons who have them. Physical disabilities seem to be inextricably linked with shame and inferiority. Thus, physical limitations produce suffering and despair much greater than the physiology of the impairment, and these feelings often affect the individual's psychologic well-being.

A disability is an undesirable thing. To think otherwise can cause unnecessary pain and embarrassment. A disability does limit an individual's capabilities. Thus, the term *disabled person* (for which the authors prefer to use *person with a disability*) refers to *an individual with impaired functioning, mental or physical, that is sufficient enough to interfere with one or more major aspects of his or her living.* A disability can be due to vision, speech, hearing, or motor impairment; birth defects; disease; or accident. An impairment limits mobility or mental functioning, but it is societal attitudes that make people handicapped.

REFERENCES

Apton, A. A. *The Handicapped.* New York: Citadel Press, 1959.

Beckett, S. *Proust.* London: J. Calder, 1965.

Bitter, J. A. *Introduction to Rehabilitation.* St. Louis: C. V. Mosby, 1979.

Brantman, M. What happens to insurance rates when handicapped people come to work? *Disabled USA.* Washington, DC: President's Committee on Employment of the Handicapped, 1978.

Burdett, M., and Frohlich, B. *The Effect of Disability in Unit Income.* Washington, DC: Social Security Administration, 1977.

Buscaglia, L. C. (Ed.). *The Disabled and Their Parents: A Counseling Challenge.* Thorofare, NJ: Charles B. Slack, 1975.

Childs, G. B. Is the work ethic realistic in an age of automation? In Peters, H., and Hansen, J. C. (Eds.). *Vocational Guidance and Career Development.* New York: Macmillan, 1971.

Cull, J. G., and Hardy, R. E. *Adjustment to Work.* Springfield, IL: Charles C Thomas, 1973.

Deutscher, M. Adult work and developmental models. In Peters, H., and Hansen, J. C. (Eds.). *Vocational Guidance and Career Development.* New York: Macmillan, 1971.

Florian, V. Employer's opinions of the disabled person or a worker. *Rehab Couns, 22:* 38–43, 1978.

Friedman, E., and Havighurst, R. *The Meaning of Work and Retirement.* Chicago: University of Chicago Press, 1954.

Haj, F. *Disability in Antiquity.* New York: Philosophical Library, 1970.

Hinshaw, D. *Take Up Thy Bed and Walk.* New York: G. P. Putnam's Sons, 1948.

Koestler, F. A. *The Unseen Minority.* New York: American Foundation for the Blind, 1976.

Koestler, F. A. *Jobs for Handicapped Persons.* New York: The Public Affairs Committee, 1980.

Koshel, J. J., and Granger, C. V. Rehabilitation terminology: Who is serving the disabled? *Rehab Lit, 39:* 102–106, 1978.

Lofquist, L. H., and Dawis, R. V. *Adjustment to Work.* New York: Appleton-Century-Crofts, 1969.

McDaniel, J. W. *Physical Disability and Human Behavior.* New York: Pergamon Press, 1970.

Nathanson, R. B. The disabled employee: Separating myth from fact. *Harvard Bus Rev, 57:* 101–110, 1979.

Obermann, C. E. *A History of Vocational Rehabilitation in America.* Minneapolis: T. S. Denison, 1965.

President's Committee on Employment of the Handicapped. *Affirmative Action for Disabled People: A Pocket Guide.* Washington, DC: U.S. Government Printing Office, 1982.

Roe, A. *The Psychology of Occupations.* New York: John Wiley & Sons, 1956.

Rubin, S. E., and Roessler, R. T. *Foundations of the Vocational Rehabilitation Process.* Baltimore: University Park Press, 1978.

Super, D. A. Developmental self concept theory of vocational behavior. In Osipow, S. H. (Ed.). *Theories of Career Development.* New York: Appleton-Century-Crofts, 1968.

Vash, C. L. *The Psychology of Disability.* New York: Springer, 1981.

Weber, M. *The Protestant Ethic and the Spirit of Capitalism.* New York: Scribner, 1930.

Weinberg, N., and Sebian, C. The Bible and disability. *Rehab Couns Bull, 23:* 273–281, 1980.

Weissman, H. Absenteeism, accidents of rehabilitation workers. *Rehab Rec, 6:* 15–17, 1965.

Wolfbein, S. L. *Work in American Society.* Glenview, IL: Scott, Foresman, 1971.

Wright, B. A. *Physical Disability: A Psychological Approach.* New York: Harper & Row, 1960.

Yuker, H., Campbell, W., and Block, J. Selection and placement of the handicapped worker. *Ind Med Surg, 29:* 419–421, 1960.

Additional Readings

Allan, W. S. *Rehabilitation: A Community Challenge.* New York: Wiley, 1958.

Appleby, J. A. *Training Programs and Placement Sources: Vocational Training and the Placement of the Severely Handicapped.* Salt Lake City: Olympus, 1978.

Bitter, J. A. *Introduction to Rehabilitation.* St. Louis: C. V. Mosby, 1979.

Bowe, F. *Handicapping America: Barriers to Disabled People.* New York: Harper & Row, 1978.

Carling, F. *And Yet We Are Human.* London: Chatto and Windes, 1962.

Ellis, F. K. *No Man Walks Alone.* Westwood, NJ: Revell, 1968.

Fitts, W. H. *The Self Concept and Performance.* Nashville, TN: Dedi Wallace Center, 1972.

Fitts, W. H. *The Self Concept and Self-Actualization.* Nashville, TN: Dedi Wallace Center, 1971.

Grossman. V. *Employing Handicapped Persons: Meeting EEOC Obligations.* Washington, DC: Bureau of National Affairs, 1980.

Hanman, B. *Physical Capacities and Job Placement.* Stockholm: Nardisk, 1951.

Hunt, P. *Stigma: The Experience of Disability.* London: Dublin, 1966.

Koestler, F. A. *Jobs for Handicapped Persons.* New York: The Public Affairs Committee, 1980.

Leviton, S. A., and Taggert, R. *Jobs for the Disabled.* Baltimore: Johns Hopkins University Press, 1977.

Pieper, J. *Leisure: The Basis of Culture.* New York: Pantheon Books, 1952.

President's Committee on Employment of the Handicapped. *The Law and Disabled People.* Washington, DC: U.S. Government Printing Office, 1980.

Spiegal, A. D., and Podair, S. (Eds.). *Rehabilitating People with Disabilities into Mainstream Society.* Park Ridge, NJ: Noyes Medical, 1981.

Weisgeber, R. A., Dahl, P. R., and Appleby, J. A. *Training the Handicapped for Productive Employment.* Rockville, MD: Aspen, 1980.

Wright, G. N. *Total Rehabilitation.* Boston: Little, Brown, 1980.

Wylie, R. C. *Self Concept.* Lincoln: University of Nebraska Press, 1961.

Chapter 2

THE NATURE OF THE PROBLEM

Individuals concerned about and committed to equal opportunities for persons with disabilities must guard against accepting and perpetuating clichés such as "I'm not prejudiced" and "I treat all people the same."

Even the most liberal individuals do not treat all people the same. As painful as it may be to admit, everyone is *for* or *against* someone or something based on prejudice. To pretend otherwise merely perpetuates problems. For instance, some parents firmly believe that children of one sex are better than those of the other or favor one child more than another. Unless prejudice is recognized, discriminatory behavior is likely to stand uncorrected. Recognition is the first step toward minimizing unfair treatment and maximizing fair treatment.

BRIEF REVIEW OF RELATED LITERATURE

Numerous studies have shown commonalities in the social and physical conditions of people who have disabilities and the psychologic reactions and negative attitudes toward them. In addition to negative conditions, however, there are also positive ones. Consistent with the authors' stated spiral approach to learning, a few of the many studies that impressed them as being insightful are presented along with their own less pedantic discussion.

Seminal work focusing on different sources of negative attitudes toward people with disabilities (Mussen and Barker, 1944; Raskin, 1956; Gellman, 1959; Wright, 1960; Roeher, 1961; Siller, 1963) showed that attitudes determine the treatment of an individual; in turn, treatment shapes the individual's personality. Each source cited clearly pointed out that negative societal attitudes toward a person with a disability produce devastating results. Such attitudes are seen in avoidance, pity, segregation, and overprotection, as well as other behaviors. Thus, negative attitudes are a main deterrent to the rehabilitation of people with disabilities.

There are some fairly well-prescribed, informal role expectations of persons with disabilities. It is not enough to have a disability; an individual must also *behave as though* he or she has one. The person with a disability is expected to grieve the loss of his or her body part or function, which reflects the value that persons without disabilities place on their own body parts or functions. (Dembo, Leviton, and Wright, 1956; Sussman, 1969; Kutner, 1971; Thorenson and Kerr, 1978). Individuals who reject the "suffering role" are likely to be verbally or physically punished. Interestingly, guilt is also attached to being able-bodied (Wright, 1960; Siller, 1963). Atonement generally manifests itself in people's contributions to charitable activities for those with disabilities.

The uneasiness that characterizes the interaction between persons without disabilities and those who have disabilities often represents fear of the unknown. Fritz Heider (1944) and Donald Hebb (1946) noted that persons in unfamiliar situations become anxious and confused. Certainly, encountering someone who has a disability represents an unfamiliar situation for those who do not have disabilities. Human bodies with missing pieces or individuals whose movement deviates from the norm tend to cause fearful and negative reactions in nondisabled observers. The lack of factual information about a disabling condition facilitates anxiety and withdrawal (English, 1971; Anthony, 1972). Feelings of repulsion and discomfort are felt when people who do not have disabilities come in contact with persons who have certain visible disabilities, e.g. skin disorders, amputations, body deformities, and cerebral palsy (Richardson et al., 1961; Siller, 1963; Safilios-Rothschild, 1968). This is referred to as *aesthetic-sexual aversion.* Related to this concept is Paul Schilder's (1935) concept of *body image,* which states that seeing a person with a physical disability causes discomfort because there is incongruence between an expected "normal" body and the actual perceived body that does not fit the expectation. This may lead to the fear of losing one's physical integrity.

Central to the rehabilitation process is how a person adjusts to his or her disability. The terms *adaptation, coping, mastery,* and *adjustment* have been used at various times to identify the process of handling disabilities, with *adjustment* being the most utilitarian term (Russell, 1981). Franklin Shontz (1978) traced the various theories of adjustment over the past three decades and divided them into three categories: (1) *person oriented,* (2) *socioenvironmental,* and (3) *integrative.* Something of value can be found in each of these approaches.

Person-oriented approaches consist of behavioral adjustment, e.g. classical conditioning and operant conditioning, and mental adjustment (individual stages of internal processes of adjustment). Although many writers (for example, Davis, 1963; Fink, 1967; Kerr and Thompson, 1972; Kubler-Ross, 1969; Shontz, 1978) have traced mental adjustment to disabilities through stages that range from shock to acceptance, few empirical data support these stages-of-adjustment theories. Even so, a large number of practitioners have found stages useful, mainly for conceptualizing processes through which persons with disabilities learn to accept their conditions. As Eileen Nickerson (1971) observed, adjustment to a disability means being able to function satisfactorily within the limits imposed by it; or, as Donald Linkowski and Marilyn Dunn (1974) concluded, acceptance of a disability is related to a positive self-concept.

Socioenvironmental approaches focus on factors that are external to the person with the disability; that is, the attitudes of other persons and the physical barriers they erect must be overcome if the person with a disability is to adjust in a socially functional way. Part of this adjustment requires abandoning or readjusting what Talcott Parsons (1951) called the *sick role* and Gerald Gordon (1966) called the *impaired role.* Some people adjust by hiding their disability. Erving Goffman (1963) called this *passing.* Ultimately, adjustment to socioenvironmental conditions means that instead of ignoring or hiding his or her disability, a person utilizes social and environmental resources to live a productive life.

Kurt Lewin (1935) and Lee Meyerson (1955) exemplified the *integrative approaches* to adjustment to disabilities. From their perspectives, adjustment is relative to the individual and his or her external forces. Specifically, factors such as age, emotional maturity, nature of physical barriers, religious beliefs, and previous coping experiences interact to affect the type of adjustment. Strategies used in the rehabilitation plan should, integrative theorists believe, relate to as many relevant approaches as possible.

Based on the studies reviewed, it should be evident that the task of understanding and abating negative attitudes is formidable. However, it is not impossible or unmanageable. Above all else, helpers who are well-informed, well-trained, and optimistic are needed.

ATTITUDES AND BEHAVIOR

Because human beings are creatures of culture, attitudes, feelings, and values make objective thinking difficult. However, behaviors, not attitudes, create the major problems in human relations. There are many laws against discriminatory behavior, but there are none against prejudicial attitudes. Human rights activists maintain that it is not what people think about those with disabilities that hurts or helps them but how people act out those thoughts. Some individuals act out their prejudices by denying people with disabilities adequate education, jobs, and housing. Because popular writings and the news media have focused on black-white conflicts and confrontations, prejudice involving other groups is inadequately reported or not reported at all.

Prejudice is not limited to color. There is prejudice against social classes, women, and many other groups. In the long list, there is prejudice against people with mental and physical disabilities. The following statement was made by a blind black man: "I think that disabled people want the same rights as blacks—human rights. I want to be able to go any place I want to go. I want to be able to go to any school. I want to be able to go to any public place. I want to be able to go to any restaurant" (Galloway, 1981, p. 189).

Prejudice is a conclusion drawn without adequate knowledge or evidence. It can multiply and spread to areas that are unrelated to the initial object of concern. The bigot blames others for various social misfortunes: floods, high taxes, inflation, wars, and, interestingly, bigotry. Such prejudgments are easier to make than objective judgments, which require more energy, knowledge, integrity, and time. In their efforts to make expedient decisions, bigots react to concepts rather than to people.

To abate prejudices, people must know their own strengths and weaknesses, understand how people become prejudiced, and empathize with the many groups that are targets of discriminatory behaviors. In short, they must understand not only their own beliefs and behavior but also the beliefs and behavior of others. People usually get back the kind of human relations they give. Acceptance fosters acceptance, and rejection brings rejection. Because each individual's personality reflects his or her intrapersonal and interpersonal experiences, some personalities can be described as ugly and stunted, while others are beautiful and dynamic.

Effective human relations result when each individual accepts and respects the differences of others. This basic principle is frequently taught but less frequently practiced. Whether positive or negative, social behavior spreads in a contagious manner. Unfortunately, only a few people living in heterogeneous environments realize that their differences are assets that provide them with an opportunity to learn from others. Many people waste the major portion of their lives rejecting potential friends who look different. Kate Hoffman (1981), a female born without one hand and "normal" in every other aspect, certainly knows how it feels to be physically different: "I became increasingly less popular till seventh grade, when I totally withdrew after the spring dance. I remember it well. Everyone was pairing off, and the popular kids dated the popular kids. I was an outsider, I was not invited. By that time, it was very, very clear that I was totally at the bottom of the social caste" (p. 29).

Americans are exposed daily to mass media programs that characterize this nation as a country dominated by physically able people. Citizens with disabilities who accept this exaggerated view of the United States become willing parties to a prophecy that fulfills itself; they become losers by default. When this happens, individuals without disabilities maintain their positions of power and pass on the socially myopic prophecy from one generation to the next. For these and other reasons, prejudice against people with disabilities is one of the most pressing human relations problems in today's society. Such prejudice is found in neighborhoods, schools, and jobs, and it comes from two main sources: the values and attitudes people learn from others, and the tensions and 'frustrations that are experienced while trying to cope with others, especially strangers.

A social attitude is a degree of readiness to behave in a given manner toward an object or situation. Much could be added to this definition to make it more scientifically precise, but it is adequate for this discussion. There are three implications of this definition for the chapters that follow:

1. A social attitude is a *degree of readiness.* . . . This is a vague statement. However, if it is thought of as the ability to perceive certain objects and situations, and the quickness to respond, motivation to respond, and experience in responding, then *degree of readiness* can stand the test of further scrutiny. An example of this process is provided by a teacher who experiences anxieties growing out of the thought of having to teach children with disabilities.

2. A social attitude is a degree of readiness to behave *in a given manner.* . . . An attitude is not an overt response. It is a response, to be sure, but an implicit or mental one. Therefore, an attitude is a readiness to act, *not* an act itself. The crucial human relations question that arises here, then, is "Under what conditions does an attitude elicit overt expression?"

   Even the most general answer to this question must include at least two variables:

A. *An attitude is likely to result in overt expression in direct proportion to rewards and in inverse proportion to punishments.* Behavior cannot always be predicted on the basis of whether it will be rewarded or punished. A weakly held attitude will produce action if the gratification for doing so is great enough.

B. *Overt behavior is likely to result when there is a degree of readiness.* Some individuals act out their attitudes, no matter how negatively the community reacts to their behavior. These individuals become martyrs for various causes, such as those of citizens with disabilities or women. On the other hand, some individuals cannot, under any circumstances, muster sufficient readiness to act out their attitudes. They say, "I know what I should do, but I can't." Technically, the degree of readiness must rise and resistance must lower to a crucial point in order for attitude to result in action. There are thresholds at which the degree of readiness (perception, motives, and response) must be sufficiently developed and the situation must be sufficiently rewarding for at least part of the attitude to result in overt behavior.

Overt behavior can mean anything, from making marks on an attitude questionnaire to dying for a cause. It is generally assumed in psychologic experiments that when most variables in a situation are held constant, the degree of action taken toward an object is a function of motivation, the desire to achieve a goal. Although this assumption may be correct in most instances, there is more to the degree of readiness than motivation. There is also a *response system*—the means used to achieve the goal. For example, two individuals, *X* and *Y*, may be equally motivated to succeed in getting children with disabilities into their youth clubs, but the response of *X* is to wait for applicants to call, while *Y* tries to obtain the names of prospective members. In a similar manner, two state legislators may be equally motivated to enact barrier-free housing legislation, but the behavior of one involves only a verbal response, whereas the other writes bills. Thus, there are talkers, doers, and talkers who are doers.

3. A social attitude is a degree of readiness to behave in a given manner *toward an object or situation*. Here, *object* and *situation* are used in the broadest senses. *Object* refers not only to individuals but also to their beliefs. Within this definition, any group of people or their behavior is considered socially significant and may become embodied in social attitudes. A social attitude toward people with disabilities, then, is a degree of readiness to behave in a given manner toward some perceived aspect of them. Whether this readiness will result in overt behavior is determined by certain conditions internal and external to the individuals involved. This is the

basic foundation for dealing with the problem of how social attitudes toward people with disabilities are formed.

People Learn to Dislike People

There are four hypotheses about attitudes that are now generally accepted: (1) Attitudes are learned; (2) attitudes are learned mainly from other people; (3) attitudes are learned mainly from other people who have high or low prestige for a particular individual; and (4) once attitudes have been learned, they are reinforced.

The first three hypotheses focus on the perception of social objects and the development of motivational and response systems appropriate for these perceptions; the fourth hypothesis suggests that attitudes are difficult to change.

1. Attitudes are learned.

Attitudes are learned; they are not innate. A mother talking about her child's prejudice against children with disabilities said: "Tina has always played with well children. She never plays with crippled children. I didn't have to teach her that." She reflects the assumption that powerfully held attitudes, such as disability prejudices, are part of an individual's inherent being. The mother apparently believed that she did not have to teach her daughter to discriminate against children with disabilities. There is evidence to the contrary.

Antidisabled attitudes have been detected in children as young as three years old (Gellman, 1959; Roeher, 1961; Weinberg, 1979). However, studies have shown that even these attitudes are not very well developed in most children until age ten or eleven. Young children begin to use hate words before they fully understand their connotations. Social scientists have documented thousands of cases illustrating that attitudes are learned. Tina's mother believed that Tina knew instinctively not to associate with "crippled" children, but her third-grade son suggested other reasons for the attitude: "Mother told me not to play with them [children with disabilities] because they are sick. . . . I had a crippled friend in school. I liked him, but Mother didn't want me to play with him." The mother had taught her children to reject children with disabilities.

Once negative attitudes are learned, children can be very cruel to peers with disabilities. They mock them and in the process either break them down or steel them to their impairments. One can walk onto almost any playground where large numbers of children gather and hear them taunting others for their physical disabilities—simulating crossed eyes, mocking slurred or stammering speech, and pantomiming epileptic seizures. It is not that children want to be cruel but that they want to be in with the in-group, just as their parents do. Much like their ancestors during the 1692 witch trials in Salem, they must have their sport.

It is not just what people without disabilities do to people with disabilities that constitutes the problem. There is a pecking order, or rank order of preference, among people with disabilities. Doe West (1981), who must spend some of her time in a wheelchair, described prejudice from within:

> If I meet a disabled person and I'm not in the chair and we're talking and I say, "Yeah, we disabled people . . . ," they sort of look at me and think, she doesn't look very disabled—she must have epilepsy or she must have a learning disability or diabetes, or something. And then as we're talking later and I say, "Yeah, you know, when I'm in the chair . . . ," they say "When you're in the *chair?*" I get this ambivalent feeling from disabled people in terms of—well, God, you're a lucky stiff; you can get out of the chair. And sometimes I'll meet anger or bitterness at the fact that I can get out of the chair. And it hurts me, because they don't understand the seriousness of my own disability. [P. 176]

The most insidious prejudices are negative attitudes directed toward groups of people. They take the form of assumptions or generalizations about all or most members of a particular group ("You know how *those* people are!"). Such in-group versus out-group hostility threatens the very existence of this nation. People are employed, housed, married, and buried with one major criterion in mind: group affiliations. The behavior, customs, and habits of out-group people are labeled *strange* and *inferior.* Most aspects of growing up with a physical disability add to the probability of societal rejection.

The learning of attitudes is seen when adults change their commitments as they move into situations in which new attitudes are more functional—for example, when they join a club or move into an "exclusive" neighborhood. Thus, new attitudes are part of a wide range of adjustment devices that every human being acquires. Attitudes of acceptance must be learned in much the same manner that people learn to reject people. It is hypothesized by many writers that most American children are taught to reject rather than accept people who are culturally and physically different. In the insightful words of Carl Jung (1968): "We still attribute to the other fellow all the evil and inferior qualities that we do not like to recognize in ourselves, and therefore have to criticize and attack him, when all that has happened is that an inferior soul has emigrated from one person to another. The world is still full of *betes noires* and scapegoats, just as it formerly teemed with witches and werewolves" (p. 65).

Researchers have noted that as children grow older, they tend to forget that they were instructed in attitudes by their parents (Horowitz and Horowitz, 1938). Around the age of ten, most children regard their attitudes toward people with disabilities as their own. Seldom do they recall having been coached by their parents. *Attitude amnesia* develops, and elaborate rationalizations are presented to account for the learned attitudes, with the result that most people believe that they came by their attitudes "naturally."

2. Attitudes are learned mainly from other people.

Most attitudes are learned from other people. As ego deflating as it may be to accept, it is a fact that few people invent their attitudes. An attitude is a complex perceptual invention, and most people are not perceptual inventors. For example, "That man has paraplegia, and, therefore, he is inferior to me," is a seemingly simple perception, but it is a straightforward attitude that includes the man *and* his label and, therefore, requires considerable rationalizing. Individuals who perceive persons with paraplegia as inferior have to think beyond individuals with paraplegia, who may be adequate by almost every objective standard, in order to define the group of *persons with paraplegia* as inferior.

The superiority or inferiority of a group (as contrasted to that of an individual) is not obvious; not many casual observers can perceive significant group differences. To illustrate, the existence of physical disabilities as a social problem is by no means obvious. Most people simply cannot think of liking or disliking physical disabilities *per se* but only of liking or disliking particular disabilities, e.g. the loss of eyesight, hearing, or use of legs. Before an attitude can be formed about an object, something must be perceived as its characteristic. Because most people are not very adept at inventing new ways (or even old ways) of perceiving the world, there seems to be a sound basis for believing that attitudes, like most things, are invented by a few and used by many.

There are other reasons for assuming that attitudes are learned largely from other people. Autobiographies and case histories illustrate that an individual's attitudes toward disabilities tend to be those of his or her relatives, sex group, peers, office mates, school group, region, religion, and nationality. Certainly, some attitudes are developed independently of significant others, but significant others are the foremost determinants of most social attitudes. Thus, the tendency of individuals to hold the same attitudes toward disabilities as the people with whom they interact is so consistent as to make independent acquisition unlikely. This does not necessarily mean that individuals learn their attitudes about disabilities only from the individuals or groups with whom they live, but it certainly suggests the importance of relatives, friends, and social institutions.

Some people will ask, "Is it true that people hold the same attitudes as those with whom they live simply because they are all exposed to similar conditions?" In other words, "Do people learn the same attitudes independently simply because they all have the same experiences? —Of course not. Although many people may look at the same phenomenon, they depend on a few "important" people to tell them what they have seen. Consequently, stereotyped attitudes toward various persons with disabilities are found among people who have had no contact with them. Furthermore, it has been found that initial attempts to change negative social attitudes through personal experience are not always successful.

The unlikelihood that individuals will invent attitudes for themselves, the correlation of their attitudes with those of the people with whom they live, and the low level of correlation between attitude and personal experiences—all of these factors point to the conclusion that attitudes are learned from other people. However, attitudes are not learned from just anyone, which leads to the third theory of attitudes.

3. Attitudes are learned mainly from other people who have high or low prestige.

Investigators have been testing this hypothesis for several decades. In a typical experiment, subjects respond to one or more attitude scales. Then they are told the attitudes of 98 percent of the nation's leading educators, of certain authorities, or of the majority of their own reference group on the same scales. Later, they are retested with equivalent tests. In most cases, the retest scores move significantly in the direction of the educators, authorities, and peers, leading inevitably to the conclusion that most people tend to match their attitudes with persons or groups important to them who have high prestige.

There are, of course, exceptions. Some individuals will not shift their attitudes to match those of an admired person if the attitude attributed to the latter is diametrically opposed to theirs. There is, nonetheless, a strong tendency for people to reinterpret their role models' statements in line with their own views rather than admit the models are wrong. "The press distorted his views," a son replied when asked about antidisability quotes attributed to his father, whom he worshipped.

The second part of the hypothesis is that people tend to adopt attitudes opposite to those of groups with low prestige. Such attitudes are likely to be held for one of two reasons: (1) Certain groups may have low prestige for people because they have rejected those people, who adopt attitudes opposite to theirs as a means of rejecting them in turn; or (2) certain groups are poor role models for people, and, thus, the people elect not to imitate them.

4. Once attitudes have been learned, they are reinforced.

If one assumes that the first three theories are correct, the initial formation of attitudes is the result of a desire to be like individuals who are held in high esteem. Once formed, however, an attitude may serve various other motives. For example, although most persons in a community learn negative attitudes toward people with disabilities from their friends, the attitudes of some persons center on economic motives. Most individuals, for instance, initially adopt antidisability attitudes in order to conform to social pressures but maintain those attitudes in order to exclude qualified job competitors with disabilities.

The economic motives that reinforce attitudes are relatively obvious. Clearly, in the short run, it is economically advantageous for one group to keep another group out of certain kinds of work, to deny them adequate legal protection in bargaining for their labors, to keep their aspirations low, or even on occasion to exterminate them. The questions that economic interpretations of social attitudes fail to answer, however, are "Why are repressive methods used against one group but not another?" and "Why are certain attitudes enforced even to the point of national disaster?" Some critics observe that as a nation, America seems to be willing to waste the human resources of people with disabilities.

Group prejudices are expressed in terms of *stereotypes,* false images of out-groups. Some stereotypes are given a typical verbal expression, such as "Cripples are pushy," "Deaf people are lazy," "Amputees are sneaky," or "Poor handicapped people are trashy." These images are clearly false, but they trigger the premature social and psychologic deaths of the people so labeled. In most instances, these images can be destroyed only after the prejudiced person has had a positive experience with a person in the stereotyped group. However, it is likely that a positive experience will only cause the prejudiced person to discount its general significance by saying, "That person is different, exceptional, not like the others." That is, people tend to refence their prejudices to exclude a few token members of the oppressed group.

In casual contacts with the handicapped, normals tend to measure them against the stereotype, and such contacts reinforce common stereotypes. An example may help to demonstrate this process. Recently, a number of typical skiers observed a blind skier coming down the slope. They spoke about him and his "amazing feat." They commented on how "truly remarkable" that he could have the courage and fortitude to do what must be exceptionally difficult for a person with no eyesight. From the tone of their comments, it was clear that they did not perceive this person as any *ordinary* blind person. The sighted skiers did not question their stereotypes of the blind as physically inept. Instead, they confirmed the stereotype by classifying this skier as an exception to the rule—as "amazing." [Bogdan and Biklen, 1981, p. 18]

How Attitudes Are Formed

There are several ways in which attitudes are formed. Being aware of these processes will better enable people to alter their negative attitudes. Some popular ideas about how attitudes are formed have been refuted in scientific experiments.

Attitudes are seldom formed by logic.

It is very difficult to find circumstances in which attitude change has come about as a result of logical argument or additional information (Wilson and Alcorn, 1969; Siperstein, Bak, and Gottlieb, 1977). When students in classroom experiments are confronted with logic or new information, they do not tend to change their attitudes. For example, racist students who receive intensive instruction in anthropology do not as a rule abandon their belief in innate racial differences. Instead, they give nonracist answers on tests in order to get passing grades. Individuals who register changes in attitude because of such information consistently fail to maintain the new attitudes as the prestige of the person presenting the logical arguments or imparting the information decreases. Therefore, not simply *what* is said but also *who* says it are important variables influencing whether an argument or information will change attitudes. Bankers and real estate developers influence housing patterns for citizens with disabilities more than college professors and factory workers.

There is the general finding that attitudes acquired by logical argument are not acted out very logically (Hafer and Narcus, 1979). For example, a college student's attitude toward people with disabilities may become more tolerant during a course in vocational rehabilitation but show very little carry-over into the job. In fact, some vocational rehabilitation trainees adopt what they perceive to be "correct" answers in order to get a diploma but revert to polar attitudes and behaviors when they are employed as rehabilitation counselors. There is not only little evidence that important attitudes are changed by logical information inputs but even considerable evidence that a great amount of information, particularly on controversial topics, actually hardens or freezes whatever attitude is already in the making.

Techniques such as an exceedingly emotional religious appeal or a relatively unstructured workshop focusing on physical disabilities often are more effective than highly structured scientific lectures. Elaborate conferences and professional seminars with "experts," situations in which opposing interests are presented in great detail, tend to produce little shift in attitude but instead add to the confusion about what attitude should be taken. The unqualified assumption that information will improve attitudes in one way or another is based on the questionable assumption that what is true and what is desirable are one and the same.

Important attitudes are seldom influenced by logic because in most cultures, including this one, logic is valued as a *means* but seldom as an *end* of life. The desired end tends to be some visible sign of success, and when the choice is between logic and success, success generally prevails. This is not to imply that most people want to seem illogical. On the contrary, most people would like to project an image of being very logical, but not if such an image will cause them to fail to achieve certain goals, especially economic ones. In some settings, little prestige accrues to individuals who associate with persons with disabilities.

The power of logic (and information) can easily be tested by following these simple steps: (1) Select an individual who is fairly neutral; (2) determine an attitude toward disabilities that he or she holds with considerable strength but which happens not to be based on logic and fact; (3) objectively and unemotionally try to alter his or her attitude by pointing out the illogical aspects of it; and (4) observe the effect. This exercise is likely to illustrate that logic and information have little to do with attitude formation. There are, however, at least two special instances in which this may not be the case. Attitudes may be formed by logic and information if the attitude to be formed or changed does not conflict with motives more powerful than the desire to be logical or if the individual in whom the attitude is to be formed or changed is one of those rare persons for whom "having it right" is more important than "having it his or her own way."

Attitudes are seldom formed as a function of intelligence.

In this day of loose and careless logic, it has been claimed that some people become radicals (or liberals) because they are more (or less) intelligent than those who become conservatives. Studies investigating intelligence and attitudes have shown correlations between intelligence and liberalism or conservatism ranging from low positive correlation to no correlation at all. There is little scientific support for attributing attitudes to intelligence (Katz, 1960). Interestingly, there is a tendency for people to believe that those who share their values are intelligent and that those who do not are stupid.

Ignorance leads people without disabilities to assume that they are superior to those with them. Nondisability is thus equated with high intelligence, while *disability* becomes synonymous with *low intelligence*. Persons engaging in such assumptions have not learned that (1) all people are of the same genus and species; (2) there are more differences within groups than among them; and (3) apparent group differences are largely attributable to environmental conditions, training, and opportunities.

Attitudes are seldom formed by personal experience.

It is often heard that integration of the handicapped would become a way of life if people of the various groups would only live together. Placing bodies together is not enough. One factor that reduces the importance of personal experience on attitude formation is the tendency of people to perceive and remember only what they are socially and psychologically prepared to see and recall. A person's friends predetermine not only how he or she reacts to a given stimulus but indeed whether he or she perceives it in the first place. Consider, then, the difficulty of changing the attitude of persons without disabilities toward those with them by getting them together, if those without are prepared to see only negative characteristics in people with disabilities.

A second factor that may reduce the importance of personal experience in shaping attitudes is the possibility that personal experiences may actually reinforce the negative attitudes that they are supposed to change. Prejudiced persons will not develop a favorable attitude when they interact as neighbors with individuals having disabilities if the behavior of the newcomers fits their existing stereotypes about people with disabilities. It is difficult for many social reformers to accept the fact that some members of groups actually reinforce the very attitudes that the reformers are eager to eradicate, i.e. some people with physical disabilities *are* behaviorally disconcerting. Judith Myers (1969) gave an illustration:

> The child's arm flailed, her head wobbled, and her eyes rolled. Before her, on the school recreation table, were the sickening shambles of a lunch. The table had been crowded around by many children. Now every one of them had beat a retreat and clustered again at a safer distance, to watch and even cruelly to mimic the helpless youngster rooting so dreadfully in her food. . . . Bits of cookie, sandwich, fruit littered the table, and the little girl gagged like a little beast. [P. 59]

Does all of this mean that personal contacts are entirely without value? —Certainly not. Negative attitudes toward people with disabilities can be formed or changed by personal experience if (1) the attitudes are not in conflict with more powerful motives, (2) the experience is carefully selected to represent people with disabilities in the best possible light, (3) the persons who are to experience changed attitudes are prepared to experience the best in the situation, or (4) the attitude involves perceptions that are so simple as to be obvious examples of empirical contradiction.

New attitudes toward people with disabilities can be learned if such experiences with them are rewarding, providing that more punishing experiences do not follow. When a couple is ridiculed by parents, peers, and others for moving into a housing unit largely occupied by persons with disabilities, they are less likely to associate with persons with disabilities, even friendly ones.

SUMMARY

Being against someone or something is not necessarily a prejudice. When based on facts, an attitude opposing someone or something is a *bias*, which does not violate democratic principles. For example, an individual is not behaving prejudicially if she concludes after interacting with a neighbor who has a disability that she does not like him. It is also important to note that not all prejudices are harmful or negative. Some, such as clothing preferences, are both harmless and a source of amusement to others. Prejudicial attitudes can support a group rather than oppose it. Black, Brown and Red Power advocates, for instance, state that they are for their people and not against other groups. These individuals are not interested in integration.

The most insidious prejudices are negative attitudes directed toward groups of people. They take the form of assumptions or generalizations about all or most members of a particular group. Being identified with an out-group adds to the probability of societal rejection of individuals with disabilities.

NOTE TO HELPERS

Efforts to bring about attitudinal and behavioral changes can and often do result in strong resistance to those changes. Alvin Zander (1950) outlined several reasons for this resistance:

1. *Resistance to change can be expected if the change is not clear to the people who are going to be influenced by the change.* Most people want to know exactly what they must do in order to help persons with disabilities. It is not enough to say, "The change is because of new laws" or "It's the right thing to do."

2. *Different people will see different meanings in the proposed change.* There is a tendency for people to see in proposed changes the things they want to see, i.e. workers with disabilities may see equal opportunities, while workers without disabilities may see "reverse discrimination." Complete information can be distorted just as easily as incomplete information, especially if the persons to be changed are insecure.

3. *Resistance can be expected when individuals in power positions are caught between strong forces pushing them to make the change and strong forces opposing the change.* If trying to bring about change, the individual or group must be able to show that there is a greater payoff for the organization to make the change rather than not make it. Little energy should be spent trying to destroy opponents' reputations.

4. *Resistance can be expected to increase to the degree that the persons in the organization influenced by the change (rank and file workers) have pressure put on them to change and decrease to the degree that these*

same persons are involved in the nature or direction of the change. It is true that behavior can be legislated or mandated, but it is also true that forcing people to accept persons with disabilities can be a fleeting victory for the organization and persons with disabilities. Change is almost always accepted and institutionalized in a non-destructive manner when the decision-making process is shared. However, ultimately, someone must be responsible for carrying out the change.

5. *Resistance may be expected if the change is made on personal grounds rather than impersonal requirements or sanctions.* After the individuals to be affected by the change have had a chance to discuss it, if they still do not want to make it, then it is not prudent for the administrator in charge to say, "I think we should do this." Who really cares what he or she thinks? A better approach is, "This change is consistent with this organization's equal opportunity/affirmative action objectives." The change should be grounded in organizational objectives and commitments.

6. *Resistance may be expected if the change ignores established group norms.* There are formal as well as informal ways changes are made within organizations. An effective change will neither ignore old customs nor abruptly create new ones. For example, if it is an informal custom for new workers to be given certain work spaces or schedules, then new workers who have disabilities should be given these spaces or schedules, too.

In summary, co-workers are likely to accept persons with disabilities when the newcomers prove that they are basically the same as persons without disabilities. Anyone who wishes to alter the status quo of organizations and positively influence the quality of life for people with disabilities would be well advised to heed Zander's warning.

REFERENCES

Anthony, W. A. Societal rehabilitation: Changing society's attitudes toward the physically and mentally disabled. *Rehab Psychol, 19:* 117–126, 1972.

Bogdan, R., and Biklen, D. Handicapism. In Spiegel, A. D., Podair, S., and Fiorito, E. (Eds.), *Rehabilitating People with Disabilities into the Mainstream of Society.* Park Ridge, NJ: Noyes Medical, 1981.

Davis, F. *Passage Through the Crisis: Polio Victims and Their Families.* New York: Bobbs-Merrill, 1963.

Dembo, T., Leviton, G. L., and Wright, B. A. Adjustment to misfortune: A problem of social psychological rehabilitation. *Artificial Limbs, 3:* 4–62, 1956.

English, R. W. Combatting stigma toward physically disabled persons. *Rehab Res Practice Rev, 2:* 1–17, 1971.

Fink, S. L. Crisis and motivation: A theoretical model. *Arch Phys Med Rehab, 48:* 592–597, 1967.

Galloway, D. Quoted in Roth, W. E. *The Handicapped Speak.* Jefferson, NC: McFarland, 1981.

Gellman, W. Roots of prejudice against the handicapped. *J Rehab, 40:* 4–6, 1959.

Goffman, E. *Stigma: Notes on the Management of Spoiled Identity.* Englewood Cliffs, NJ: Prentice-Hall, 1963.

Gordon, G. A. *Role Theory and Illness: A Sociological Perspective.* New Haven, CT: College & University Press, 1966.

Hafer, M., and Narcus, M. Information and attitude toward disability. *Rehab Couns Bull, 23:* 95–102, 1979.

Hebb, D. O. On the nature of fear. *Psychol Rev, 51:* 259–276, 1944.

Heider, F. Social perception and phenomenal causality. *Psychol Rev, 51:* 358–374, 1944.

Hoffman, K. Quoted in Roth, W. E. *The Handicapped Speak.* Jefferson, NC: McFarland, 1981.

Horowitz, E. L., and Horowitz, R. E. Development of social attitudes in children. *Sociometry, 1:* 301–338, 1938.

Jung, C. G. *Civilization in Transition,* vol. 10. Princeton, NJ: Princeton University Press, 1968.

Katz, D. The functional approach to the study of attitudes. *Pub Opinion Q, 24:* 163–204, 1960.

Kerr, W. G., and Thompson, M. A. Acceptance of disability of sudden onset of paraplegia. *Paraplegia, 10:* 94–102, 1972.

Kubler-Ross, E. *On Death and Dying.* New York: Macmillan, 1969.

Kutner, B. The social psychology of disability. In Neff, W. S. (Ed.). *Rehabilitation Psychology.* Washington, DC: American Psychological Association, 1971.

Lewin, K. A. *A Dynamic Theory of Personality.* New York: McGraw-Hill, 1935.

Linkowski, D. C., and Dunn, M. A. Self-concept and acceptance of disability. *Rehab Couns Bull, 18:* 28–32, 1974.

Meyerson, L. Somatopsychology of physical disability. In Cruickshank, W. M. (Ed.). *Psychology of Exceptional Children and Youth.* Englewood Cliffs, NJ: Prentice-Hall, 1955.

Mussen, P. H., and Barker, R. G. Attitudes toward cripples. *J Abnorm Soc Psychol, 39:* 351–355, 1944.

Myers, J. M. The linneth on the leaf. In Kvaraceus, W. C., and Hayes, E. N. (Eds.). *If Your Child Is Handicapped.* Boston: Porter Sargent, 1969.

Nickerson, E. T. Some correlates of adjustment by paraplegics. *Precept Mot Skills, 32:* 11–23, 1971.

Chapter 3

WHO ARE THE DISABLED?

A social activist agreed to ride to a meeting with a friend who had a disability. They found the place of the meeting but had difficulty locating the parking spaces reserved for persons with disabilities. Finally, after fifteen minutes of circling around the parking area, they decided to ask a security guard for directions to the parking spaces. Addressing the social activist, he gave clear directions. Somewhat embarrassed, she thanked the guard and quickly added, "The parking space is for her" (pointing to her friend). The guard smiled and said, "It looks to me like both of you need it."

EXAMPLES OF PHYSICAL DISABILITIES

A cursory review of statistics pertaining to people with disabilities in the United States is overwhelming. There are approximately 25 million adults with disabilities between the ages of sixteen and sixty-four; between the ages of three and twenty-one there are approximately 10 million persons with disabilities who are impaired enough to require special education in the public schools. One-fourth of all American citizens sixty-five years of age and over have disabilities. Frank Bowe (1980) put the various statistics into a chilling perspective:

> Of the 15 million disabled Americans between the ages of 16 and 64 who are not institutionalized more than 7.7 million are either out of the labor force or unemployed. Most have given up, and they have because they cannot obtain the education they need for employment, cannot get a job training in many fields, cannot secure transportation to and from work, and cannot find suitable places to live. Our failure to invest in these people and their potential has forced them into dependency programs. [Pp. 8–9]

These overlapping statistics give estimates of 36 million to 50 million Americans with disabilities, and the number is growing as the population ages. People with disabilities comprise the nation's largest open minority group—anyone may join at any time. Disability is not restricted to any race, ethnic group, gender, age, social class, religion, or geographic boundary. Whatever the cause or nature of his or her disability, each person is an individual who must overcome barriers to his or her functioning as an integral member of the community.

In 1980, the number of people with chronic conditions resulting in some type of severe disability was as follows:

5.5 million had arthritis and rheumatism.
5.2 million had heart ailments.
2.9 million had impairments of the back and spine.
3.1 million had hypertension.
2 million had disorders of the nervous system.
2.5 million had impairments of the lower extremities or hips.
1.6 million had diabetes.
1.4 million were visually impaired.
1.4 million had asthma.
700,000 had hearing impairments.

If the people who have mild disabilities are included in these statistics, the numbers are even larger:

20 million Americans have hearing problems.
200,000 Americans are deaf.

Table 3.I shows a few specific disabilities.

DIABETES. Actually, *diabetes* is the name of two diseases that have the same sign, excessive urination: *diabetes mellitus* and *diabetes insipidus*. Diabetes mellitus is the more common of the two, and neither of the diseases can be cured. Most of the estimated 10 million persons in America with diabetes have diabetes mellitus. It is characterized by abnormal amounts of sugar in the blood and sugar in the urine. Too much sugar in the blood and urine causes continuous thirst, passing of large amounts of urine, and loss of weight and strength. Untreated persons with diabetes may have

TABLE 3-I

PERSONS WITH ACTIVITY LIMITATION DUE TO CHRONIC CONDITIONS, 1980

Activity limitation, sex and age	Number of persons limited in activity (millions)	Selected chronic condition[1]								
		Arthritis, rheuma-tism	Heart conditions	Hyper-[2] tension	Diabetes	Asthma with or w/o hay fever	Impairments of back/spine	Impairments of lower extremity or hip	Visual impairments	Hearing impairments
		Percent of persons limited in activity because of specified condition								
All degrees of activity limitation										
Both sexes, all ages	31.4	17.5	16.4	9.9	5.2	4.6	9.2	8.0	4.5	2.4
Under 45 years	10.2	5.4	4.3	3.3	2.3	9.0	13.9	10.7	3.3	2.9
45–64	10.4	20.0	19.7	13.2	6.4	3.0	9.9	7.2	3.1	1.7
65 and over	10.8	26.5	24.5	13.1	6.7	1.8	4.0	6.4	6.9	2.6
Male, all ages	15.5	11.0	18.0	7.7	4.3	4.4	9.1	9.0	4.6	2.8
Female, all ages	15.9	23.7	14.7	12.1	6.0	4.7	9.2	7.1	4.4	2.0
Limited but not in major activity										
Both sexes, all ages	7.6	12.8	8.5	6.8	3.6	7.0	8.9	11.7	4.8	3.8
Under 45 years	3.9	4.4	3.4	2.8	1.9	10.7	11.1	14.9	3.8	3.4
45–64	2.2	16.5	13.1	11.2	5.3	3.9	9.2	9.7	3.2	3.7
65 and over	1.5	29.6	14.8	10.7	5.6	*2.1	2.6	6.2	9.9	4.9
Limited in amount or kind of major activities										
Both sexes, all ages	15.7	19.9	15.5	10.6	5.2	4.7	10.7	6.6	3.5	1.9
Under 45 years	5.1	6.6	4.1	3.5	2.9	9.2	16.5	7.4	2.9	2.7
45–64	5.4	22.6	18.6	14.3	6.4	3.1	10.6	6.1	2.5	1.1
65 and over	5.2	30.2	23.5	14.0	6.3	1.8	4.9	6.3	5.0	2.0

TABLE 3-I (continued)

PERSONS WITH ACTIVITY LIMITATION DUE TO CHRONIC CONDITIONS, 1980

Activity limitation sex and age	Number of persons limited in activity (millions)	Selected chronic condition[1]								
		Arthritis, rheumatism	Heart conditions	Hyper-[2] tension	Diabetes	Asthma with or w/o hay fever	Impairments of back/spine	Impairments of lower extremity or hip	Visual impairments	Hearing impairments
		Percent of persons limited in activity because of specified condition								
Unable to carry on major activity										
Both sexes, all ages......	8.1	17.1	25.5	11.5	6.5	2.0	6.5	7.4	6.1	2.0
Under 45 years.........	1.2	3.3	8.5	4.2	*0.9	*2.5	11.6	10.9	3.4	*1.7
45-64..............	2.8	17.6	26.9	12.7	7.3	2.3	9.1	7.3	4.2	*1.2
65 and over.........	4.1	20.7	29.3	12.8	7.4	1.7	3.3	6.5	8.1	2.6

Covers civilian, noninstitutionalized population. Based on unpublished data from the National Health Interview Survey, National Center for Health Statistics, U.S. Department of Health and Human Services.

[1] Ninth Revision of the International Classification of Diseases used for coding in 1979.

[2] Includes all cases of hypertension regardless of other conditions.

*Figure does not meet standards of reliability or precision.

Source: National Center for Health Statistics, U.S. Department of Health and Human Services.

attacks of boils, carbuncles, and other infections. They also risk decreased blood circulation and gangrene. Treatment mainly consists of insulin and proper diet. Mild cases of diabetes mellitus can be controlled by diet alone.

Diabetes insipidus results from injury or disease of the posterior lobe of the pituitary gland. Treatment is with pitressin, an extract from the posterior lobe of the pituitary gland. Victims of diabetes are more likely women than men, nonwhites than whites, and low-income people than middle– and upper-income people.

CEREBRAL PALSY. This is a condition caused by injury to the cells in the motor area of the brain. Approximately 700,000 persons in the United States have cerebral palsy. The damage to the brain, which cannot be repaired, may occur at any time during a person's life, and it can be the result of various things, including disease, accidents, or stroke. Contrary to popular opinion, all persons with cerebral palsy are not of low intelligence. In fact, people with cerebral palsy exhibit the total spectrum of intelligence, with most of them having normal and above-normal intelligence.

There are five major conditions of cerebral palsy: spastic, athetoid, ataxia, tremor, and rigidity. Almost 90 percent of the conditions are spastic and athetoid. The muscles are tense and frequently contracted in spastics, resulting in considerable difficulty controlling body movements. The athetoid condition is characterized by involuntary and uncontrollable movement. Sometimes the symptoms are mixed, e.g. a person who is mainly spastic in movement may be athetoid in some. Ataxia is a condition of imbalance and distorted sense of direction. Persons with this condition may stagger and fall frequently. Tremor appears as trembling hands, feet, arms, and legs. Rigidity is characterized by stiff and rigid muscles. Persons with this condition have difficulty moving their muscles to new positions.

Cerebral palsy is also classified by the portion of the body affected: If one limb is affected, it is called *monoplegia;* partial or complete paralysis of two limbs on the same side of the body is called *hemiplegia; diplegia* refers to both upper or both lower limbs; *paraplegia* is complete paralysis of the lower half of the body; and *triplegia* refers to paralysis in three limbs (both legs and one arm or both arms and one leg)

Physical therapy is used to train the large muscles (legs and arms) so that individuals can walk and move about better; occupational therapy trains the smaller muscles (hands, fingers, and toes) so that they can take care of other needs, such as eating, writing, and dressing. Speech therapists help individuals with impaired speech muscles to speak more clearly.

MUSCULAR DYSTROPHY. This disease attacks the voluntary muscles, especially those that control arm and leg movements. The progression of the disease ranges from very slow to rapid deterioration. As with cerebral palsy, the mobility of persons with muscular dystrophy ranges from slight restrictions to immobility. Currently, the major symptom is weakness attributable to muscle deterioration. There is no effective treatment for muscular dystrophy, but many persons with the disease are able to live active, productive lives. More than 200,000 people in the United States have muscular dystrophy. Most victims inherit the disease.

CYSTIC FIBROSIS. This disease is also hereditary. It is characterized by abnormally thick mucus that forms plugs in body organs, thereby negatively affecting their operation. For example, the mucus may obstruct air passages and interfere with breathing. There is no cure for the disease; it is treated with antibiotics, enzymes, and sometimes surgery. There are 13,000 to 30,000 persons in the United States with cystic fibrosis.

MULTIPLE SCLEROSIS (MS). This disease attacks the brain and spinal cord. The cause of MS is unknown, and there is no cure for it. Symptoms include blurred vision, paralysis of the arms or legs, poor balance, and stiff muscles. The disease may last many years or just a few, and it is terminal. Rest and antidepressants are the treatment. Approximately 500,000 people in the United States have multiple sclerosis.

ARTHRITIS. Although not publicly feared as much as the preceding conditions, arthritis, an inflammation of the joints of the body, is a major disability. There are many different types of arthritis. Some types are caused by injury; some by infections; some by aging; and some by unknown causes. The major forms of chronic arthritis are (1) rheumatoid arthritis, (2) osteoarthritis, and (3) gout.

Rheumatoid arthritis, the worst form, can develop at any age, although it usually begins in middle age. It causes swelling and pain, stiffening of the joints, and crippling. In most cases treatment includes a well-balanced diet, ample rest, exercise, heat, and pain-relieving medication. There is no cure for rheumatoid arthritis, but most of the persons who have it are able to function well.

Osteoarthritis is the result of wear and tear on the joints. It is a common ailment among persons over fifty years of age. However, it is seldom crippling. It is characterized by a painful back, sore knees, and aching fingers. The treatment is similar to that used for rheumatoid arthritis.

Gout is caused by crystals of uric acid deposited in the tissues around joints, particularly in the feet, causing swelling and pain. Treatment consists of limiting the amount of protein in the diet and taking drugs to eliminate the uric acid. Gout is not curable, but it is controllable. Approximately 5 million Americans have some form of arthritis.

Some people have more difficulty adjusting to their disabilities than others. Usually their slowness to adjust reflects opportunities, societal norms, and prejudices rather than innate abilities.

CHILDREN

John Gliedman and William Roth (1980) described children with disabilities as the "unexpected minority." In most schools, these physically visible yet academically invisible children are characterized in terms of the following disabilities: visual impairments, hearing impairments, speech impairments, and orthopedic impairments.

VISUAL IMPAIRMENTS. Approximately one-fourth of all school children require special eye care, and more than 1 million Americans suffer from glaucoma, which sometimes leads to blindness. Visually disabled students exhibit many symptoms, including the inability to see objects and words at a distance, inflamed and watery eyes, squinting or frowning, difficulty in distinguishing colors, and redness or swelling of eyelids. All students with and without signs of defective vision should be examined by an eye specialist.

Partially sighted students, those with vision of 20/70 or less after correction, need not be hindered in the regular classroom if some adjustments are made, e.g. positioning the desks so that students who have limited vision receive sufficient light, locating their desks near the front of the room, covering or repainting highly reflective surfaces, scheduling course assignments so that there is ample time for students to rest their eyes when close visual tasks are required, using books with large type, encouraging the use of soft, dark lead pencils, and allowing partially sighted students to make oral reports if they have a great deal of difficulty with written reports.

HEARING IMPAIRMENTS. Hard-of-hearing students can be taught in regular classrooms if they can lip-read or if electronic hearing devices are available, and if their speech is not severely retarded. The major problem in the education of people with total loss of hearing, especially those who have never heard speech, is retarded speech. This also is a problem for many students with hearing loss. Children with total hearing loss are best taught in special classes because their physical disability requires extra attention (Katz, Mathis, and Merrill, 1974).

Deafness in adults generally is traceable to early childhood. Because progressive deafness is a gradual process, it usually is not noticed until hearing loss is too severe to be corrected. For this reason, early detection is imperative. Physiologic causes of deafness include malnutrition, bad teeth, inflammation of the middle ear, hardened impacted wax in the ear, and automobile collisions. Within the classroom, teachers should be alert to the following student symptoms of loss of hearing: failure to respond to direct questions, faulty pronunciation of common words, watching others and following their movement, frequent requests to repeat words, earaches, discharge from ears, and persistent mouth breathing.

SPEECH IMPAIRMENTS. Individuals with speech impairments comprise the largest group of students with disabilities. Generally, a speech defect is any acoustic variation from an accepted speech standard so extreme as to be evident to the speaker, confusing to the listener, or unpleasant to either the speaker or the listener. The list of speech impairments is lengthy and includes stuttering, stammering, lisping, and balking. One of the most common, improperly diagnosed, and inadequately treated perceptual and speech disabilities is dyslexia. Although more than 2 million American children suffer from dyslexia, fewer than 10 percent are involved in reading clinics. Dyslexic students' directional perception is distorted: They reverse letters, words, and numbers, so that *d* becomes *b,* *some* becomes *mose,* and *63* becomes *36.* With proper diagnosis and treatment, dyslexia, as well as speech problems that have no organic origin, can be corrected in elementary school.

ORTHOPEDIC IMPAIRMENTS. Orthopedically impaired students are the most visible because they require immediate school adjustments in transportation, furniture, entrances, elevators, and toilet facilities. Fewer than 1 percent of all schools make the needed adjustments. Part of the reason is finance, but part of it also is desire. Unfortunately, many people erroneously believe that all children with orthopedic disabilities are intellectually handicapped.

Major causes of orthopedic handicaps are infantile paralysis, rheumatic fever, brain injury, spastic paralysis, and tuberculosis. More than 5 million school-aged children suffer from some form of brain damage as a result of poor prenatal care, injury during birth, or a blow to the head after birth. To date, few teachers have been adequately prepared to work with children who have orthopedic impairments.

The list of students with other physical disabilities is both long and alarming—the malnourished, the underutilized, and those suffering from allergies, cardiac disorders, diabetes, tuberculosis, and other diseases. These conditions did not begin in school, and, sadly, few will end there. Substantial "catching up" must be done to achieve educational parity for the more than 10 million children with disabilities in the United States. Because of inadequate educational services, many children with disabilities currently attend private or public schools outside their own school districts. The Education for All Handicapped Children Act of 1975 (PL 94-142) was designed to alter these negative conditions.

PL 94-42 defines *handicapped children* as mentally retarded, hard of hearing, deaf, speech impaired, visually handicapped, seriously emotionally disturbed, orthopedically impaired, or other health-impaired children or children with specific learning disabilities who by reason thereof require special education and related services.

In terms of children with disabilities who are sufficiently impaired to warrant special services, the ratios in the major categories are as follows (Henderson, 1978):

Speech impaired	30 per 1000
Hard-of-hearing	6 per 1000
Crippled	5 per 1000
Partially sighted	5 per 1000
Blind	3 per 1000
Deaf	2 per 1000

A growing number of school and community programs are being established to prevent children with disabilities from becoming handicapped.

WOMEN

As a prelude to the feminist movement in the Church, Jeanne Richie (1971) wrote: "It is my conviction that the problem of women's status in American society is urgent. . . . I believe that the systematic subordination of women in America must be ended. . . . I believe also that this is a question which should be of particular concern to our churches, since they are so heavily dependent on the support of women and since few institutions so systematically deny women full participation" (p. 225).

Numerous writers (Greenblum, 1977; Fine and Asch, 1981; Thurer, 1982; Vash, 1982) have statistically documented the occupational plight of women with disabilities: Approximately 70 percent of women with disabilities and 30 percent of men with disabilities are unemployed. This means that males with disabilities are more likely than females with disabilities to be referred to vocational schools and on-the-job training. Women with disabilities are more likely to be underemployed than men with disabilities, and they are less likely to be college educated. They earn substantially less than their male peers and have lower levels of disability coverage and insurance benefits.

Women with disabilities are mainly employed in traditional "female" jobs that have low salaries. In 1976, the mean weekly wage for women in rehabilitation programs was $63, compared with $112 for their male peers. Only 2 percent of the women earned $200 or more per week at the end of their rehabilitation program, compared with 10 percent of the men (Thurer, 1982). However, as women with disabilities become more socially and politically active, many of the leadership roles once held by men with disabilities are being shared with women with disabilities, to the point that in isolated instances, males with disabilities are crying "Reverse discrimination," as employers fill their handicapped quotas with females instead of males.

Paula Franklin (1977) pointed out that women with disabilities are socially disadvantaged because they are less likely than other women to marry, are more likely to divorce, and have more absent spouses (separated, divorced, or widowed) than men with disabilities. There is a larger percentage of female heads of households with disabilities than male heads of households with disabilities.

Ruth Mauer (1979) suggested that the disadvantages begin early in life; females with disabilities have lower self-images than their male peers. The females in her study were more likely than males to identify with a story character with a disability; most males identified with the character without the disability. Social forces push a disproportionate number of women to behave like their negative stereotypes. This should not be surprising. Although there are relatively few socially successful models for people with disabilities in general, there are even fewer for females with disabilities.

THE ELDERLY

Since the 1880s, the increase in the number of births, advances in medical technology, development of more disease-fighting drugs, and better understanding of the functions of the body and diseases have led to increases in life expectancy. According to the National Center for Health Statistics, the life expectancy for women is approximately seventy-eight years; for men, it is seventy years. The elderly population in the United States is estimated at 25 million and growing. The United States Bureau of the Census projects that by the year 2000, there will be more than 30 million elderly persons in the United States. (A person in America is defined as being elderly at age sixty-five.)

As crude as it may sound, it is true that the body is a machine and that, as with all machines, it becomes less functional with age. Brittle bones, less stamina, and decreased range of motion are but a few of the factors that can cause the elderly to become less active. However, there are older individuals who are physically active, and their mental abilities are sharp enough to allow them to manage their own affairs. Conversely, some individuals who are younger than sixty-five show many of the classic signs attributed to the elderly—physical frailty and slow mental process. Workers differ greatly in their mental and physical characteristics at all ages (Botwinick, 1977), although as a group, older workers tend to be more heterogeneous than other workers (Butler, 1975).

Elderly persons with disabilities have a double disability. They must struggle to survive two types of stigma—one associated with normal physical limitations and the other associated with being placed in a category that presupposes great intellectual limitations. (*See* Chapter 5 for how this principle relates to ethnic minorities with disabilities.) Robert Atchley (1980) explained the overall stigma attached to old age.

> By far, the most important aspect of the stigma of old age is its negative disqualifying character on the basis of their age; older people are often relegated to a position in society in which they are no longer judged to be of any use or importance. Unless they have special talents or skills, or can afford to support themselves well in retirement, older people often find that the stigma of old age limits their opportunities. Like most "expendable" elements in society, many older people are subjected to poverty, illness, and social isolation. [P. 16]

Elderly people with disabilities may be the most discriminated-against persons in America. In terms of productivity, very little is expected of the elderly in general, and almost nothing is expected of those with disabilities (Butler, 1975; Rosen and Jerdee, 1976). Even sadder than this is the fact that very few attempts are made to provide them with ways of maintaining their self-esteem. Most views of the elderly are quite morbid; their lives are perceived as being over, and all that needs to be done is for them to lie down and close their eyes.

AND MEN, TOO

Generally, the most important factor for men who have disabilities is whether they are still able to perform physical tasks. In many instances, cosmetic devices do little more than hide the disability, while the functional limitations remain. Siller (1963) and Zola (1982) documented that artificial limbs and other protheses create an illusion of no disability but that these devices often do little to curb negative attitudes and behavior toward physical disability. For men who perceive themselves as heads of households and general leaders and protectors of their families, adjustment to disability is particularly difficult.

As a growing number of females are receiving treatment equal to that of men, they, too, are becoming concerned with tasks rather than physical appearance (Thurer, 1982).

OTHER GENERAL CHARACTERISTICS OF THE DISABLED

Although a seminal study by Sar Leviton and Robert Taggert (1977) is somewhat dated, still valid are their observations that individuals with disabilities have a great distance to travel to reach full equality in America: They are less educated and less employed and receive less pay than people without disabilities.

EMPLOYMENT. According to Richard Burkhauser and Robert Haveman (1982), 17 percent of Americans report some type of disability. There is danger in basing projections on self-reports of medical conditions, but these results have been corroborated in other studies. Besides, scientific studies are not needed to get a feeling for the economic plight of people with disabilities. With respect to the effect of disabilities on employment, over one-half of the self-perceived disabled believe their disability presents limitations severe enough to prevent them from working on a regular basis or working at all. Almost one-fourth of the population sampled believe that their disability created a need for a change in occupations or caused them to be restricted to part-time employment.

EDUCATION. Over one-third of the persons classified as having severe disabilities have less than eight years of formal education, compared with less than 10 percent of people without disabilities.

Part of this disparity is attributable to the fact that ethnic minorities and persons considered to be in the lower socioeconomic strata of society comprise a larger percentage of persons with disabilities than whites and middle– and upper-income persons (Bowe, 1980). Numerous studies have indicated that ethnic minorities and lower-income individuals have lower educational achievement than nonminorities and affluent persons.

ECONOMIC STATUS. Because the population with disabilities has a disproportionate number of women and ethnic minorities, two groups that have historically been paid less than white males, it is not surprising that a large proportion of this population is classified as low income. Disability is more prevalent among women than among men; almost 20 percent of American women have some degree of disability, compared to slightly more than 15 percent of the men. Blacks and other ethnic minorities comprise 12 percent of the total working population, but they make up 15 percent of the population with disabilities and over 18 percent of persons with severe disabilities.

A BROADER VIEW

Everyone has limitations. Fears and phobias create limitations that restrict activities and functioning of individuals who possess them. For example, a person who has difficulty functioning satisfactorily in high places may be unable to ride in an airplane or on a Ferris wheel or work on high-rise construction jobs. Most people who are afraid of large bodies of water not only avoid jobs such as commercial fishing and coast guard service but also limit the type of recreational activities in which they participate, e.g. they avoid water skiing, swimming, boating, and pleasure fishing. These types of limitations can comprise *emotional disability,* or *the inability of an individual to function adequately in a work, play, or social setting because of barriers imposed by internal fears.*

Weisgerber, Dahl, and Appleby (1980) argued that

all of us are limited in some way — perhaps limited in strength or agility, in vision or hearing, in mental powers or emotional stability, or simply in how well we spend or carry out other aspects of our daily lives. Certainly no one is perfect. There is enormous variability among human beings, in

part due to cultural and social influences, but also because of greater
factors, nutritional deficiencies and illness, the advance of age, accidents
or even welfare. [P. 3]

Emotional disabilities represent only one small area of limitations
that humans experience. When entering the realm of formal social activities, all persons experience some degree of *social disability,*
or *the inability to relate adequately to a social setting because of either
social deprivation or inadequate knowledge of appropriate social protocol.*
For example, an individual may refuse to attend dinner parties
because he or she does not know "proper" table etiquette.

There may be some overlapping and merging aspects of social
and emotional disabilities. An individual may refuse to go to
dinner parties because of inadequate table graces and also because
of his or her fear of crowds. This indicates both social and emotional disability. People who have social or emotional disabilities
may experience limitations in certain areas of functioning, but
this does not mean that they cannot do well in other areas.

BARRIERS

The Architectural and Transportation Barriers Compliance
Board (1979) succinctly described the following barriers that confront people with disabilities: (1) architectural barriers, e.g. steps
and entrances; (2) attitudinal barriers, e.g. pity and sympathy;
(3) educational barriers, e.g. texts not in Braille and lectures not in
sign language; and (4) informational barriers, e.g. uncaptioned
films and unraised letters in elevators). In addition, barriers may
be in occupation, e.g. unemployment and underemployment;
transportation, e.g. buses too high from the ground to be boarded
safely; housing, e.g. only public, institutional housing for persons
with disabilities; and recreation, e.g. turnstiles in theaters and
overly gravelled paths in parks.

SUMMARY

Much of the data presented in this chapter indicates that people
with physical disabilities, as well as those who have social and
emotional disabilities, have been treated as less than first-class

citizens. They often are denied gainful employment, and because of attitudinal and architectural barriers, they are denied educational opportunities that would allow them to maximize their human potentials. Prejudice and unrealistic views of people with disabilities have caused them to be relegated to a social purgatory. In spite of the many disappointments they have encountered, they continue to demand respect, insist on working when and whenever they are allowed, and persist in their efforts to live independently. With such drive and determination, it is likely that people with disabilities will someday be free of the stigma of being "different."

NOTE TO HELPERS

Although a considerable amount of statistics is presented in this chapter, it is important never to lose sight of the *individual* who has a disability. As Carl Jung (1957) said:

> It is not the universal and regular that characterize the individual, but rather the unique. He is not to be understood as a recurrent unit but as something unique and singular.... At the same time man, as member of a species, can and must be described as a statistical unit; otherwise nothing general could be said about him.... This results in a universally valid anthropology or psychology ... with an abstract picture of man as an average unit from which all individual features have been removed. But it is precisely these features which are of paramount importance for understanding man.... The individual, however, as an irrational datum, is the true and authentic carrier of reality, the concrete man as opposed to the unreal ideal or normal man to whom the scientific statements refer. [Pp. 16–20]

It is imperative that those involved in helping people who have disabilities avoid labeling, stereotyping, generalizing, categorizing, and rationalizing the unique human being who defies reduction and simplification. Scientific data and theories have their place and have provided varied and invaluable heuristic tools to use as helpers, but data and theories should be discarded when they cease to assist in understanding and helping individuals with disabilities.

REFERENCES

Architectural and Transportation Barriers Compliance Board. *About Barriers.* Washington, DC: U.S. Government Printing Office, 1979.

Atchley, R. C. *The Social Forces in Later Life.* Belmont, CA: Wadsworth, 1980.

Botwinick, J. Intellectual abilities. In Birren, J. E., and Schaie, K. W. (Eds.). *Handbook of the Psychology of Aging.* New York: Van Nostrand Reinhold, 1977.

Bowe, F. *Rehabilitating America.* New York: Harper & Row, 1980.

Burkhauser, R. V., and Haveman, R. H. *Disability and Work: The Economics of American Policy.* Baltimore: Johns Hopkins University Press, 1982.

Butler, R. N. *Why Survive? Being Old in America.* New York: Harper & Row, 1975.

Fine, M., and Asch, A. Disabled women: Sexism without the pedestal. *J Sociol Soc Welfare, 8:* 233–248, 1981.

Franklin, P. A. Impact of a disability on family structure. *Soc Sec Bull, 40:* 3–18, 1977.

Gliedman, J. C., and Roth, W. *The Unexpected Minority: Handicapped Children in America.* New York: Harcourt Brace Jovanovich, 1980.

Greenblum, Joseph. Effect of vocational rehabilitation on employment and earnings of the disabled: State variations. *Soc Sec Bull, 40:* 3–16, 1977.

Hamilton, K. W. Counseling the handicapped in the rehabilitation process. In Wright, Beatrice A. *Physical Disability: A Psychological Approach.* New York: Harper & Row, 1960.

Henderson, G. *Introduction to American Education: A Human Relations Approach.* Norman: University of Oklahoma Press, 1978.

Jung, C. G. *The Undiscovered Self.* New York: Mentor, 1957.

Katz, L., Mathis, S. L., and Merrill, E. C. *The Deaf Child in the Public Schools.* Danville, IL: Interstate, 1974.

Leviton, S., and Taggart, R. *Jobs for the Disabled.* Baltimore: Johns Hopkins University Press, 1977.

Mauer, R. A. Young children's response to physically disabled storybook hero. *Except Child, 45:* 326–330, 1979.

Richie, J. Church, caste and women. In Marty, M. E., and Peerman, D. G. (Eds.). *New Theology No. 8: Our Cultural Revolution.* New York: Macmillan, 1971.

Rosen, B., and Jerdee, T. H. Influence of age stereotype on management decisions. *J App Psychol, 6:* 428–432, 1976.

Siller, J. Reactions to physical disability. *Rehab Couns Bull, 7:* 12–16, 1963.

Thurer, S. L. Women and rehabilitation. *Rehab Lit, 43:* 194–197, 1982.

Vash, C. L. Employment issues for women with disabilities. *Rehab Lit, 43:* 198–207, 1982.

Weisgerber, R. A., Dahl, P. R., and Appleby, J. A. *Training the Handicapped for Productive Employment.* Rockville, MD: Aspen, 1980.

Zola, I. K. *Missing Pieces.* Philadelphia: Temple University, 1982.

Additional Readings

Cannon, J. R. *Deaf Heritage: A Narrative History.* Silver Springs, MD: National Association of the Deaf, 1981.

Guitar, B., and Peters, T. J. *Stuttering: An Integration of Contemporary Therapies.* Memphis, TN: Speech Foundation of America, 1986.

Lindemann, J. E. *Psychological and Behavioral Aspects of Physical Disability.* New York: Plenum Press, 1981.

Phillips, W. R. F., and Rosenberg, J. (Eds.). *The Physically Handicapped in Society,* 39 vols. New York: Arno Press, 1981.

Chapter 4

PERCEPTIONS

The perceptions of people without disabilities concerning the social worth of individuals with disabilities defy sweeping generalizations. Most books and articles written about the social and psychological aspects of disability indicate that societies foster contradictory attitudes toward people with disabilities. Individuals with disabilities often are seen within the same community as being good and evil, able and unable, adult and childish (Barker and Wright, 1963). The contradictions are abundant. Furthermore, subcultural attitudes toward disabilities reflect ambivalence (Harosymia, Horne, and Lewis, 1976). Some people view a disability as a sign of inferiority, while others regard it as an indication of virtue or physical fortitude. The latter view is more common in subcultures where suffering is considered a means to attaining deep understanding and wisdom.

Reflecting societal ambiguity, a person with a disability is more likely than a person without a disability to be unsure of his or her reception by others. This chapter will discuss (1) how negative perceptions of people with disabilities are formed; (2) some common negative perceptions of disabilities; and (3) several strategies for changing these negative perceptions.

HOW NEGATIVE PERCEPTIONS ARE FORMED

An old adage states that first impressions are lasting. What is there about some people with physical disabilities that causes negative images to be formed? The answer to this question points out the importance of group interaction, self-concept, and human needs. The answer is primarily culturally determined.

Appearance

Daily, man is bombarded with thousands of stimuli that prompt him to form ideas and attitudes about his surroundings, e.g. the physical appearance of some food causes him to form a perception of its taste without actually having tasted it, while the appearance of a room may cause him to form a perception of its occupants long before he has interacted with them or knows them personally. Whether perceptions are correct or incorrect is not the issue. Even if they are false, this does not alter the fact that appearance is a very important factor in attitude formation.

People with physical disabilities are not a rare phenomenon, and seldom are they as odd as they sometimes appear at first glance. However, when the effects of deafness, speech defects, blindness, and cerebral palsy distort a viewer's perception, differences are magnified, and this hides the fact that, as a group, people with disabilities are more like people without disabilities than they are different from them. A parent of a child with a disability wrote:

"My son has cerebral palsy. He cannot stand. He cannot control his hands to hold or turn the pages of a book. Nor can he hold his head still. His efforts to talk so distort his features that strangers turn away with a shudder. Yet within this misshapen body is a brilliant and sympathetic mind, a mind that has allowed my son to build for himself a satisfying life and accept his handicap with grace" (Kvaraceus and Hayes, 1969, p. 7).

Most societies place great emphasis on physical beauty. This obsession with physical wholeness and perfect physiques is called the *body beautiful obsession.* The effect of this obsession is partially measured by the numerous drugs, exercise apparatus, and books that promise the development of perfect physiques. Packaging good health has spawned multibillion-dollar businesses. Few people argue against the virtues of balanced diets, weight control, and proper exercise; however, obsession with the physique often goes far beyond being healthy. Through subtle and not-too-subtle advertisements, the message is clear: The closer individuals come to looking like Mr. Olympia or Miss America, the more they are considered all-American men and women. Conversely, the further a body deviates from these standards, the less it is to be valued.

As seen in Chapter 1, discrimination based on physique is neither a recent nor an insignificant occurrence. Since the earliest times, class and caste have included physical distinctions. The ancient Greeks believed that those with physical disabilities were inferior persons. Modern literature, comic books, television, and theater have used negative physical appearances to develop villainous characters (Weinberg and Santana, 1978; Thurer, 1980; Livneh, 1980). The deformed appearances and malevolent behavior associated with characters who have disabilities tend to foster a negative perception of people with disabilities. Of course, this is countered when characters with disabilities are endowed with wisdom and charity. Unfortunately, the characterizations are uneven. Body intactness and good health are more likely to be ascribed to good and noble characters, while physical deformity is a common trait of evil and malevolent characters.

The physical appearances of several well-known literary characters have been used not only to depict individuals with physical defects but also to imply that they have some inner or emotional defect; even their souls are bad. Captain Hook, the villainous character in *Peter Pan*, Chaucer's Summoner, and Shakespeare's Richard III—all have visible physical defects, and all are characterized as having severe emotional problems. The one-legged Captain Ahab in Herman Melville's *Moby Dick* and Doctor Frankenstein's monster are other examples. Even good characters such as Quasimoto, the Hunchback of Notre Dame, and Cyrano de Bergerac are heroes *because of* their disabilities, which repulse people. Furthermore, the presence of superintelligent or superstrong characters with disabilities perpetuates "abnormal" or "freak" images, however virtuous the individuals may be.

Comic books are much more widely read than classical literature. When children read comic books without proper guidance, they are likely to develop a strong belief that physical disabilities are inherent in evil persons. A disproportionate number of comic-book villains are physically disabled. It takes maturity and perceptual sophistication for young readers to accept characters with disabilities as ordinary people who happen to have a disability, rather than to see them as abnormal people who have negative traits that overshadow and influence every other aspect of their lives.

Persons with lupus, kidney disorders, arteriosclerosis, diabetes mellitus, and epilepsy have what have been referred to as *invisible disabilities.* Since appearance is the foremost factor in forming the initial perception of persons with disabilities, people who have disabilities that are not easily noticed are perceived as being "normal." Public attitudes vary according to the nature, severity, and prognosis of the disability. Generally, children with disabilities are better accepted by the public than adults with the same disabilities. As a group, individuals with mild disabilities have higher self-concepts than those with severe disabilities. The less visible the disability, the more positively an individual is viewed by his or her peers, or, stated another way, the less visible the disability, the more a person fits the stereotype of normality. This perception has its advantages and its disadvantages.

Frequently, social adjustment is measured in terms of an individual's ability to appear normal. In this instance, the standard of appearance is nondisability. Jo Campling (1981) told the following story of Maggie, who was diagnosed while in college as having hereditary, incurable progressive nerve damage: "I found I could bluff my way out of awkward situations by acting the part of a rather scatty dolly bird. It wasn't that I couldn't hear you but rather that I was such a feather-brained, aspiring actress that I just didn't understand what you meant. It seemed more acceptable to be a 'normal' silly butterfly than an intelligent deaf woman" (p. 34).

The same standards of judgment and behavior that apply to people without disabilities are applied to persons with invisible disabilities. This unqualified acceptance allows them to function without having to overcome additional barriers of pity, sympathy, and rejection. Like the economically poor person who didn't know that he was culturally disadvantaged until he took his first sociology course, many persons with invisible disabilities do not know the seriousness of their condition until told. Confirmation of a disability is usually accompanied by trauma—shock and sadness followed by fear and shame.

Although a disability may not be visible to the average person, the individual with it does indeed have limitations. In order to enjoy unqualified acceptance as normal persons, the invisibly disabled must, or believe they must, conceal their physical limitations. Once knowledge of their disability is known, they are likely to lose social status. Thus, like light-skinned blacks during the pre–civil rights days, many persons with invisible disabilities "pass" for persons without disabilities. In concealing their disabilities, they may aggravate them, i.e. an individual with a heart condition may attempt to do things that he should not do, or a person with diabetes may refuse to take her medication. Because of unapparent limitations, these individuals may not receive feedback that is needed for them to deal realistically with their conditions (Marenelli and Dell Orto, 1977). Of course, one could argue that many persons with obvious disabilities do not receive helpful feedback either.

Knowledge of How the Disability Occurred

The initial belief that a person with a disability is good or evil, intelligent or stupid, saved or sinful is determined in part by how the disability occurred. Most cultures are less willing to accept or subscribe to a sympathetic attitude toward a person if his or her disability occurred as a result of a socially defined foolish act, e.g. drunken or reckless driving, use of drugs, or playing Russian roulette with a handgun. In these instances, the prevailing attitudes is, "They [the persons with the disability] got what they deserved" or "They are paying for their sins." However, if an individual is born with a disability or it occurred through non-negligence, sympathy is likely to be given. However, it is empathy, not sympathy, that is needed.

There is a hierarchy of stigma associated with perceptions of physical disabilities (Olshansky, 1965). Physical disability is more readily accepted than mental disability. There is also a social class factor that influences perceptions of disabilities. A middle-class person with a mental illness is less stigmatized than a lower-class person with the same illness. There is an old saying, "If you are rich and act strange, society calls you eccentric, but if you are poor and act strange, society calls you crazy." A similar condition exists when describing societal attitudes toward physical disabilities.

Prior Knowledge of the Disability

Another way that perceptions are formed is by having prior knowledge of the subject. The more people know about individuals with disabilities, the better they are at forming accurate perceptions of the individuals' abilities and character. However, few persons without disabilities come in contact with people with disabilities. Feeling somewhat uncomfortable in the presence of individuals with disabilities, most able-bodied people avoid contact with them, even though the interaction may benefit both themselves and the other persons. Often people without disabilities avoid the contact because they do not know what to say. They fear that they may say the wrong thing, erroneously believing that there is a special language to be used when communicating with people who have disabilities.

Through contact with people with disabilities, those without them may learn that the two groups are more alike than different. Both groups have similar wants, desires, and needs. Except for the limitations imposed by disabilities, people are basically the same: They laugh, get angry, become frustrated, think dirty thoughts, and dream Freudian things. People without disabilities seldom learn that most people with disabilities are not overly sensitive about their condition. In fact, most of the sensitivity they express centers on the uneasiness of individuals without disabilities struggling to be comfortable in their presence. This calls to mind the conflicting emotions of people attending a circus freak show: They do not know whether to stare, talk, or feel guilty.

When forming an opinion based on contact with a person who has a disability, care should be taken not to overgeneralize. Just as it is important not to assume that all people who are six feet, nine inches tall are good basketball players, the behavior, good or bad, of one or a few persons with disabilities is not generalizable to all persons with similar disabilities. Yet, this is precisely the mistake that is usually made. Based on limited exposure, it is tempting to say that people with disabilities are moody or extremely self-conscious or deeply religious. These generalizations often are made after observing a sample of one.

People without disabilities must learn to view people with

disabilities as individuals and to attribute traits to them as individuals. The task is to view disabilities realistically. That is, it is important to know that disabilities produce limitations but not a different breed of human beings, alien creatures from another planet or grotesque figments from a nightmare. Whether people without disabilities will allow themselves to get close enough to persons with physical disabilities to get to know them depends to a large extent upon their own self-concepts.

One of the reasons people (even if they have a disability themselves) may feel uncomfortable around people with disabilities is a feeling of uncertainty about their own net worth. The disabled persons may be the others' mirror image, a reminder of what they can or have become, and their body image is threatened. Besides, most people fear losing their physical integrity. Profound anxiety about becoming or being handicapped plays a crucial part in the formation of prejudice against people with physical disabilities. Thus, people tend to avoid those with disabilities because they are reminded of how fragile life forms are. In reality, there is a very thin line between people without disabilities and those with them. The presence of the second group reminds people in the first that at any time they can lose the use of a leg or an arm or an eye from a variety of means—stroke, accident, disease. Consequently, people with this anxiety avoid superficial encounters (formal situations) and also nonsuperficial ones (dating and marriage) with individuals who have disabilities. Perhaps they really avoid the encounter so as not to be identified as "one of them."

Attitudes of People with Disabilities

The development of negative self-perceptions fuels a vicious circle from which few persons with disabilities can extricate themselves. They often have erroneous ideas about how they should act and what they should feel about themselves. Individuals without disabilities become aware of these notions, and most of them respond accordingly, thus fulfilling the prophecy. Alas, this is a catch-22 situation: The initial negative behavior tends to reinforce negative stereotypes. However, failure to conform to existing stereotypes may be equally hazardous to a person's social survival. Nonconforming individuals with disabilities are described as being arrogant, uppity, and hostile. There are at least five factors that affect the adjustment of an individual with a disability: (1) physical or mental impairment, (2) individual abilities, (3) disability, (4) social barriers, and (5) major life activities.

> Consider an individual who is blind (blindness caused by either congenital factors or accident or disease), partially or totally; the ability to see is affected accordingly. Here the impairment of eyes caused the inability to see. This means the individual has a visual disability. The society, say, has a negative attitude toward blindness and blind people, perhaps due to fear, anxiety, or their general inability to accommodate the blind in social settings. Such a negative societal attitude, coupled with the disability, engenders a series of obstacles or conditions—cumulatively known as the handicap—which limits a disabled person in performance of major life activities (social roles) such as occupations, recreation, marriage, and extracurricular activities (belonging to social clubs or organizations). [Seethamma and Majumder, 1981, p. 60]

Marenelli and Dell Orto (1977) suggest that adaptation, acceptance, and adjustment to physical disabilities depend to a great extent on interaction with an individual's significant others within the environment and his or her interpretation of their reactions. The basic needs of most people with disabilities are the same as those of most other people: They need love, new experience, recognition, and acceptance. Indeed, any individual's self-concept is shaped by his or her experiences centering on fulfilling these needs. The shyness shown by many persons with disabilities and their inability to function well in social settings probably reflect rejection received when trying to "fit in." Conversely, the aggressive behavior of some persons with disabilities often is attributed to their being bitter about their physical limitations. In many instances, aggressive behavior is the easiest way they can protect themselves from further rejection or misplaced sympathy.

It is normal to base perceptions of people on the way they present themselves, e.g. their stated beliefs, mannerisms, and speech patterns. Furthermore, it is highly unlikely that when forming a perception of individuals with a disability, the average person without a disability will understand why people react in certain ways to their disabilities. In other words, the person without a disability is not likely to be empathic to persons with a disability.

It seems almost too simplistic to say that the behavior of a few persons, regardless of whether that behavior is favorable of unfavorable, should not be projected to all persons. By now it should be clear that the authors of this book believe that the most humane thing that can happen to people with disabilities is to be treated as individuals of worth and dignity.

COMMON PERCEPTIONS

Most people want to know where they fit in the larger scheme of things. That is, they want to know if they are part of their community's in-groups or out-groups. People are married, hired, and included in community activities based on their group identity. Generally, persons with disabilities have low social and economic attraction and, needless to say, are in out-groups. The dominant standards of people without disabilities doom many persons with disabilities to failure, humiliation, and inferiority. Even for those who manage to emulate persons without disabilities, victory is often bittersweet and fleeting. Raymond Goldman's life illustrates this:

> At the age of 4 he was stricken with polio. Laboriously he learned to sit up, to crawl. At the age of 8 he was fitted with long leg braces. By the time he was 12, he could walk straighter and faster and tripped less frequently. At about the age of 14 he was fitted with half-leg braces and could walk better than ever. Finally, he attempted the impossible and succeeded. Contrary to the prediction of his doctor, at the age of 17 he learned to walk without braces.
>
> And yet, though he triumphed over severe difficulties, though his gait represented remarkable improvement over the years, his feeling of achievement in situations where the normal standards remained exemplary, as in contacts with girls, was abruptly replaced by the feeling of shame and dismay. ... What had been true accomplishment in terms of progress was now seen as defeat and failure because in this situation the normal standards of walking were glorified into how one *should* walk. [Wright, 1960, pp. 25–26]

People with Disabilities Are Inferior

This is a society of categorizers. People assign other people labels that place them in categories: *high income, middle income, low income, black, white, red, nonhandicapped,* and *handicapped.* Even though this society does not openly subscribe to a caste system that identifies people as being superior or inferior, it does openly subscribe to the principle that some people are more equal than others. Through words and body language people are indeed placed in categories ranging from superior to inferior. Fortunately, there is mobility within groups—low-status people can improve their situation.

By placing physical and economic barriers in the paths of individuals with disabilities, society sends messages to them that, when decoded, mean, "You are not wanted. You are not respected. You are not as good as those who are not restricted. You are, in summary, inferior." Few people without disabilities openly admit to feeling superior to people with disabilities. However, the statement, "There but for the grace of God go I," succinctly captures a thought that runs through the mind of many persons without disabilities. Humility tends to give way to personal relief when nondisabled persons see an individual in a wheelchair trying to cross a busy street or when they observe someone with cerebral palsy struggling to climb a few steps.

In addition to the feeling of pity, there is the feeling of being better than a person with a disability. This is true even though the evidence from research studies shows that publicly expressed attitudes of people without disabilities toward persons with physical disabilities seldom are negative. The fact that most people publicly state positive feelings about people with disabilities does not mean that they truly think of them as equals. The norm of this society is to tolerate and be kind to people with disabilities, for, as the saying goes, "If you can't say something nice about someone, then don't say anything." Ronald Comer and June Pillavin (1975) concluded that most Americans find it quite unnerving to admit having negative feelings toward people with disabilities.

As seen in Chapter 3, the basis for an individual's subconscious perception of a person with a disability as inferior is likely to be grounded in the fact that the words *disability* and *handicapped* imply *abnormality.* A disabled person is inferior in the minds of many people because he or she deviates from societal physical norms and often requires special assistance such as sheltered workshop employment, special toilet facilities, and reserved parking spaces. As a whole, Americans are not far removed from their pioneer ancestry, during which rugged individualism was the rule. In fact, Americans are constantly looking for new frontiers and people to conquer.

The standard by which people judge others often is how useful and independent they are. Independence is valued, and those who are dependent are condemned. One only has to say the word *welfare* in a public or private gathering to elicit a variety of not-too-complimentary terms: *lazy, shirkers, goldbricks, good-for-nothings,* and *chronic dependents.* The authors do not deny that persons with disabilities depend on some type of assistance, whether for special devices, economic assistance, or interpersonal acceptance. However, few of them are malingerers or good-for-nothings.

People with Disabilities are Totally Impaired

Consider the following statements by Frances Goldman (1978): "When I am at a restaurant with an able-bodied woman, a waitress may turn to her and say, 'What will he have?' Sometimes a stranger will walk by and pat me on the head. She will say, 'It is good to see you out.'" The manner in which most persons with physical disabilities are treated would, Goldman concluded, cause casual observers to believe them either unable to speak or retarded or both. For example, even if they have only an orthopedic handicap for which they must use a wheelchair, many persons with paraplegia are treated like imbeciles. Persons without disabilities who treat a paraplegic this way believe that a physical disability goes beyond the physical realm and contaminates all areas of the person's being, physical and psychological.

Taking the gargantuan leap from one perceived characteristic (physical disability) to other characteristics (emotional or mental problems) is referred to as the *spread phenomenon.* Of course, there are instances when an accident or a disease does indeed impair a person's intellect or emotions; however, this generally is the exception rather than the rule. People with physical disabilities are too often perceived as being totally impaired. This misperception is symbolized by a person without a disability shouting at a nondeaf person with total loss of vision in order to communicate.

People with Disabilities Are Less Intelligent

Just as few individuals will admit to feeling superior to people with disabilities, few will admit to thinking that people with physical disabilities are less intelligent than people without disabilities. However, their actions frequently expose their hidden perceptions. Generally, the severity of the disability has a bearing on the general perception of an individual's intelligence. An individual whose body is twisted and distorted by cerebral palsy is more likely to be considered retarded than a blind person or someone with one limb amputated or missing. Individuals with a speech impairment are likely to be perceived as being learning disabled. Again, the reason for these perceptions is their deviation from the amorphous norm. The more an individual's disability deviates from what society considers as physical normality, the greater the chances he or she will be perceived as being less intelligent.

There is an economically debilitating aspect in defining *adults with disabilities* as having low intelligence. Family members and friends sometimes bring arts and crafts home for them to do — cheap jewelry, leather, pottery. These are believed to be the only suitable jobs for them. Much of this "help" is given without malice, and this condescension is not without reasonable basis. There are too many unemployed and underemployed college graduates with disabilities. Even so, this does not justify behavior that diminishes the self and the opportunities for a person with a disability.

People with Disabilities Need Charity

Upon learning that a person has a physical disability, many people are overcome by images, usually of a depressed and unhappy person. In a study of social stereotyping of people with physical disabilities, Nancy Weinberg (1976) found that they were viewed as being less happy, less cheerful, and less popular than people without disabilities. It is difficult for some persons without

disabilities to conceive of happy persons with disabilities, especially if the disability is severe. Disability is viewed as not being
able to enjoy the things other people enjoy, such as physical
exercise, dating, and vacationing. In most cases, people with disabilities are able to enjoy these activities but are prematurely
prevented from doing so by well-meaning friends and relatives.

Individuals without disabilities often feel sorry for those "unfortunate people." This feeling of sorrow may lead to a feeling of
wanting to "do something" for the "handicapped." Often what is
done is dehumanizing. In many instances, people who want to
help individuals who have disabilities do not want to interact with
them. In psychological terms this is called the *approach-avoidance
phenomenon*. People without disabilities often are repelled by an
uncomfortable feeling when around individuals with disabilities
but at the same time are drawn to them out of a desire to help
them. Besides, for people who are religious, their sect probably
requires true believers to help the sick and infirm. The intention
to help the handicapped usually is a good intention. Few persons
giving charity do so to make others feel bad. However, regardless
of intent, many persons with disabilities feel degraded and inferior because they are the reason for a charity drive.

Too often, the methods and techniques that are used to raise
money for charity are degrading. These activities tend to drama-
tize the plight of people with disabilities in order to evoke feelings
of pity in potential donors. For example, by parading a child with
a severe disability before an audience, a telethon may do more
than create a charitable feeling among its viewers; it also may
create an image in their minds that the child and others like him
are totally dependent and need a handout rather than a handup.
Robert Ruffner (1982) hypothesized that because of the negative
images presented by media programs, a large percent of the viewers
feel justified treating people with disabilities as second-class citizens,
incapable of fully participating in society.

There are varying degrees of limitations imposed by a disability,
and persons with disabilities need varying degrees of assistance.
Creating an image of all or most people with disabilities as a
pathetic group damages their self-esteem and consequently does
more harm than good. It is incredible that many individuals

involved in charity activity are not aware that they actually are working against the goal they are attempting to accomplish: to raise enough money to fund projects that will assist people with disabilities to become more independent and more actively involved in the mainstream of society. Clearly, fund-raising methods that degrade and misrepresent the desires and abilities of people as a group are counterproductive.

This is not an argument for abolishing telethons and other activities to raise funds to assist the needy. Rather, it is an argument for the abolishment of activities that display persons with disabilities as totally helpless in order to evoke sympathy. The lack of a positive public image hampers the quest of persons with disabilities for social and economic integration. What the public thinks about disabilities and how it reacts to people with disabilities determine each individual's place in society.

Individuals with Disabilities Prefer
the Company of Others with Disabilities

Of course, the national perception of people with disabilities has undergone much positive change since the mid 1880s when Dorothea Dix, one of the leading social reformers of that time, fought to prevent people with disabilities from being hidden or buried in asylums so as not to come in contact with the nondisabled. Altruistically, they were sheltered from the stares and probing questions that were directed at those who were brave enough to venture among the populace. In some instances, individuals with severe disabilities were locked away in closets and cellars. This was common treatment for individuals who were mentally retarded. (To better understand the attitude of that period, it helps to know that this was the time of America's frontier expansion and that, relatedly, a person's net worth was judged by his or her ability to contribute to the expansion. Few persons with physical disabilities could clear fields, build cabins, or break wild horses.)

Currently, society does not discourage people with disabilities from being visible; however, being visible and being fully integrated into society are not always the same. They certainly are not the same in this case. Nationally, America still segregates people with disabilities from the rest of the public. Some communities place persons with disabilities in sheltered workshops that afford them little contact with other persons. When discussing housing, planners usually discuss "housing for the handicapped" instead of housing that will accommodate people with disabilities. The current trend in public housing is to make all the units completely accessible to all people. This accelerates the spread of segregated housing based on structural design, for relatively few people without disabilities are attracted to these units. Another approach would be scattered facilities, building some units to accommodate persons with disabilities and others to be utilized by persons without disabilities. It is extremely important for people without disabilities to have positive contact with people who have disabilities in an environment in which everyone is treated as individuals.

Segregation of persons with disabilities does not take on the viciousness of segregation of ethnic minority groups, although the results are the same. Of course, there is double jeopardy if an individual is disabled and a member of an ethnic minority group, and there is triple jeopardy if an individual is a female with a disability who is a member of an ethnic minority group. In summary, people with disabilities are encouraged to work, play, and live together for several reasons:

1. There is a general lack of understanding of disabilities, i.e. what persons with disabilities are capable of doing and how they feel about themselves.
2. There is the belief that individuals with disabilities have more in common with each other, regardless of their disabilities, than with other persons. On close examination, however, usually the only thing individuals with disabilities have in common is their disability.
3. There is a feeling of being uncomfortable when associating with persons with disabilities. Few people know what to do or how to react in the presence of an individual with a disability. Some people go to great lengths to avoid the uncomfortable encounter and the possibility of embarrassing themselves.
4. There is a need to protect people with disabilities. This

attitude, while well intended, produces social cripples. It is true that individuals with disabilities may experience embarrassment and degrading situations when associating with other persons, but there is a greater embarrassment: being left out.

CHANGING PERCEPTIONS OF PEOPLE WITH DISABILITIES

Much needs to be done to change America's national negative perceptions of physical disabilities. It is difficult to change most deeply rooted perceptions, and it is even more difficult to alter negative perceptions about "abnormal" people. This is true even though most physical limitations can be overcome. Donald Wilson (1970) concluded that the negative attitudes of persons with disabilities toward their disabilities, as well as the attitudes of their relatives, potential employers, and peers, are the greatest roadblocks. All persons concerned with human rights in general and the rights of people with disabilities in particular must become involved in changing these attitudes. However, the brunt of the battle must be borne by people with disabilities. By taking the lead, they clearly demonstrate to others that this is their battle. It is not easy for people who have been protected and directed most of their lives to assume responsibility for their destiny. Slowly, they are learning that only they are responsible for determining their destinies—what they will be, what hurdles they will try to clear, what they want to contest, and how they will contest it.

People with physical disabilities are uniting and taking charge of campaigns designed to gain them recognition as first-class citizens. War veterans, especially Vietnam veterans, have been very vocal about their rights. During the past decade, they have organized to protest what they consider a lack of public concern for their needs. Other persons with physical disabilities have taken note of these efforts and are beginning to unite and ask that their needs be met, too. Several steps are being taken to change societal perceptions of people with disabilities, including the following:

1. *People with disabilities are showing themselves as having power.*

Most Americans understand and respect power. They may speak negatively about those who possess it, but most strive to attain some degree of power. Even a naive person is likely to recognize that with power he or she is able to accomplish much more than without it. People with physical disabilities are seeking power to effect local, state, and national changes. Specifically, they are using ballot power to pass and implement laws that will improve their quality of life. Many minority groups—blacks, American Indians, elderly, and farm workers, to name a few—have used political leverage to further their causes. Americans with disabilities are one of the last minority groups to use political power to their advantage.

It is true that attitudes cannot be legislated, but it is also true that laws can be passed mandating equal opportunity and affirmative action for citizens with disabilities. Further, as other minority groups have discovered, passing laws is not the complete solution. Laws must be obeyed. The classic example is the civil rights laws and constitutional amendments guaranteeing equal opportunities to black Americans. It took marches and other protests to get government officials to enforce the laws and regulations.

A growing number of persons, especially persons with disabilities, are demonstrating a genuine interest in the welfare of people with disabilities. Sophisticated voters examine candidates for their views toward people with disabilities and other minorities. If a candidate is prejudiced against ethnic minorities, he or she probably is prejudiced against people with disabilities. Voters with disabilities are beginning to support actively candidates who speak out for the rights of the handicapped. One respected person in the highest places of power can get the attention of millions. The elderly found this to be true with their forceful advocate, Congressman Claude Pepper.

2. *People with disabilities are asking for more positions of authority in agencies established to assist them.*

There are a number of public and private organizations established to provide assistance to people with disabilities: vocational rehabilitation departments, leagues for the blind, Goodwill Industries, the Easter Seal Society, organizations for the visually handicapped, and many other workshops and centers. A few of these organizations and agencies are headed by persons with disabilities, and some also have a significant number of persons with disabilities on their professional staffs. Unfortunately, many agencies do not employ persons with physical disabilities in professional positions. They will take their money and provide services, but they do not employ them.

Just as it is ingrained in the minds of the public that blacks will head the Urban League and the National Association for the Advancement of Colored People (NAACP) and Jews will head Jewish organizations, the same thinking can apply to agencies servicing persons with disabilities. As they organize, people with disabilities are demanding that a greater number of executive and staff positions in rehabilitation agencies be filled with qualified persons with disabilities. When they are placed in positions of authority, two important things happen: (1) They are better able to determine their own destiny, and (2) they are placed up front, thus projecting an image of themselves as intelligent, capable people.

3. People with disabilities want more positive images of themselves in electronic medias.

Most surveys show that the major forms of entertainment for Americans are television and movies. The ability of television and movies to establish the image of groups has already been discussed. Consumers with disabilities are beginning to organize and use their collective power to demand that they be portrayed more realistically. Recently, they have begun to demand the following things from the media:

1. that people with disabilities be portrayed in films as ordinary people;
2. that more documentaries and specials portray people with disabilities as useful and fully participating citizens;
3. that television and movie producers actively seek and employ more persons with physical disabilities;

4. that whenever a television show, movie, or theatrical production portrays a person with a disability, if possible a person with a disability should fill the part;
5. that producers of commercials utilize persons with disabilities;
6. that colleges of fine arts recruit students with disabilities and train them to become actors;
7. that children's programs portray people with disabilities as ordinary human beings.

The production of children's programs that realistically portray people with disabilities is very important. Psychologists and educators are aware of how impressionable children are and how they are influenced by the visual media. Researchers Reginald Jones and Dorothy Sisk (1970) found in a study designed to trace the development of the perception of orthopedic disabilities during the formative years that, as early as age four, children become aware of physical disabilities. At five years of age they begin to view physical disabilities in negative terms and begin to refer to children with braces on their legs as "cripples."

4. People with disabilities are developing a marketing identity.

Generally, people with physical disabilities eat the same food as other people. Therefore, as advertising thinking goes, there is no need to develop advertising strategies to sell food to the physically different. This is true for most products. However, some products are enclosed in containers that are difficult for persons with physical disabilities to handle or open. Other products have labels that are difficult for a visually impaired (not legally blind) person to read, and many persons with physical disabilities have difficulty holding other products. These products are targets of selective protests.

Robert Ruffner (1982) stated that as a result of persons with disabilities not having a marketing identity, manufacturers and providers of services do not consider them a population whose business they should attempt to win. Ruffner attributes this neglect to a lack of information about disabilities, which is necessary for establishing a marketing identity. Ruffner points out that the following marketing survey questions seldom are asked about persons with disabilities: "Where do they live?" "What are their incomes?" "What do they buy, read, and watch on television?"

Currently, the little marketing that does focus on disabilities comes from industries that produce items to assist persons with disabilities, e.g. those that produce wheelchairs, braces, automobile control devices, wheelchair lifts, and hospital beds. Ironically, the marketing of these items generally is not directed at the consumers but instead at the agencies and organizations that assist them. No amount of neglect can alter the fact that people with disabilities are consumers. They spend money and deserve to be perceived as customers worth courting. Selective use of their purchasing power is beginning to give people with disabilities clout in the marketplace. When they use that clout in larger numbers, businesses will pay even more attention to them.

SUMMARY

As they accomplish the things stated above, people with physical disabilities project to the public a positive image. Already they are sending messages that they are people to be considered in almost any decision made in this country. Contrary to popular belief, the majority of persons with physical disabilities do not dislike themselves. Nancy Weinberg and Judy Williams (1978) found considerable evidence to support the view that most persons with physical disabilities do not view their disabilities as the greatest tragedy in their lives. The majority of those sampled generally considered their disability as a fact of life, an inconvenience, and sometimes a cause of frustration, but not the most terrible thing that has happened to them.

In many ways, people with physical disabilities are the country's new "niggers." They frequently are misunderstood, often despised, and seldom accepted by persons without disabilities as peers. The gravity of this situation requires attention and constructive action. It does not need any more benign neglect. Dedicated individuals are chipping away at the negative perceptions that have too long debilitated people with disabilities.

NOTE TO HELPERS

"Sticks and stones can break our bones, and words *can* socially and psychologically hurt us." What people call other people does matter. The following helpful guidelines, *Portraying Persons with Disabilities in Print*, were developed by the National Easter Seal Society.*

1. Out of respect for the uniqueness and worth of the whole individual and because a disabling condition may or may not be handicapping, use the word *disability* rather than the word *handicap*, but give reference to the person first. Make it *person/individual* with a disability or *person/individual* who has a disability. In the plural case, *persons*, *individuals*, and *people* may all be used. Avoid using the derivative word *disabled* as a labeling adjective, which implies that the person as a person is disabled, as in the expression *disabled person* or *person who is disabled*. Also avoid using *disabled* as a noun, which implies a state of separateness or total disability, as in *the disabled*.

2. Because the person is not the condition, reference to the person in terms of the condition he or she has is inaccurate as well as demeaning. Avoid, then, reference to the person as *a postpolio, a c.p., a stroke, an epileptic, a hemiplegic*, etc. Say, instead, the person who . . . *had/has polio, has cerebral palsy or c.p., had/experienced a stroke, has hemiplegia*, etc.

3. Some categorical terms are used correctly only when communicating technical information—for example, *hard-of-hearing, deaf, partially sighted*, and *blind*. More accurate choices when referring generally to persons who have disabilities of these kinds are *person/individual who has a partial hearing loss, person with a total/severe hearing loss, person who has limited/partial vision, person with total/severe loss of vision*.

4. Avoid all terms carrying negative or judgmental connotations and replace them with objective descriptions. Some examples are:

AFFLICTED BY/AFFLICTED WITH—say the person *has*.

CRIPPLE/CRIPPLED/THE CRIPPLED—say the person *with a disability/ individual with a disability caused by or resulting from/persons with disabilities*.

DRAIN/BURDEN—say *condition requiring increased or additional responsibility/person whose condition requires intensive or additional care or adjustment*.

HOMEBOUND—say *person whose ability to leave the home is limited*.

INFLICTED—say *caused by*.

INVALID (literally, not valid)—say the person *who has a disability resulting from or caused by*.

LAME—say person *with an orthopedic disability*.

*Reproduced by permission of the National Easter Seal Society, 2023 West Ogden Avenue, Chicago, Illinois 60612.

RESTRICTED TO/CONFINED TO—say *uses a wheelchair/walks with crutches.*

VICTIM—say person *who has*/person *who experienced*/person *with.*

WHEELCHAIR BOUND—say *uses a wheelchair.*

UNFORTUNATE, PITIFUL, POOR, and other such words carrying judgments; DEAF AND DUMB, BLIND AS A BAT, CRIP, FREAK, DEFORMED, and other such clichés and terms that stereotype, disparage, and offend—*No Replacements.*

5. Be careful with certain words that, if used incorrectly, can reinforce negative misconceptions of persons who have disabilities. These include:

DEFECT/DEFECTIVE—Acceptable for describing an object in error or at fault, such as a defective printout or a defective piece of equipment. Degrading and offensive when used in connection with human beings. Say problem/condition; some alternatives for *birth defect—difference in physical structure at birth,* or *lack of formation of* ( ), or *disability present at birth,* or *born with ( ).*

DIAGNOSE—Accurate only when used in connection with a condition or a disease—for example, *The condition was diagnosed as osteomyelitis.* A person is never diagnosed, but may be *found to have* or *determined to have* whatever the condition or disease may be.

DISEASE—Acceptable when referring to or classifying some causes of some disabilities—for example, polio, Parkinson's disease, meningitis—which are diseases. Misleading and inaccurate to believe or imply that persons who have disabilities are chronically ill or sick. Although a disability may be caused by a disease, the disability is not the disease itself and, therefore, can never be contagious (as is too often mistakenly thought).

NORMAL—Acceptable for referring to statistical norms and averages. Demeaning when used in reference to persons who have no disability. Say *persons without disabilities* instead.

PATIENT—Acceptable for referring to "an individual awaiting or under medical care and treatment," such as that administered in hospitals and doctors' offices. Although a few persons connected with Easter Seals may be patients, most of them are *clients* or *consumers;* none is ever a *case.*

The National Easter Seal Society summarizes what the authors believe is an excellent overview for individuals who want to portray people with disabilities correctly:

1. Emphasize the uniqueness and worth of all persons rather than differences between persons.
2. Keep the individual in perspective; avoid emphasizing the disability to the exclusion of individual qualities and achievements.
3. Show individuals with a disability doing something independently or for someone else—for example, as parents, community leaders, teachers, business owners, etc., and as participants and decision makers in their own programs of rehabilitation.

4. Show persons with disabilities in least restrictive environment, participating in activities in a manner that includes them as part of society and interacting with persons without disabilities in ways that are mutually beneficial rather than in those that foster the attitude of "one of them" vs. "one of us."
5. Depict the *typical* achiever as well as the superachiever.
6. Be consistent but compliant when referencing titles retained by organizations such as Crippled Children's Services, Office of Handicapped Individuals, and Spastics Society.

REFERENCES

Barker, Roger G., and Wright, Beatrice A. The social psychology of adjustment of physical disability. *Psychological Aspects of Physical Disability.* Washington, DC: U.S. Government Printing Office, 1963.

Bryan, Willie V. *The Effects of Short Term Individual and Group Counseling on the Self Concept of Physically Handicapped Workers in a Sheltered Workshop Setting.* Unpublished doctoral dissertation. University of Oklahoma, 1973.

Campling, Jo. (Ed.). *Images of Ourselves: Women with Disabilities Talking.* Boston: Routledge and Kegan Paul, 1981.

Comer, Ronald C., and Pillavin, June A. As others see us: Attitudes of physically handicapped and normals toward own and others groups. *Rehab Lit, 36:* 206–221, 1975.

Goldman, Frances. Environmental barriers to sociocultural integration: The insiders' perspectives. *Rehab Lit, 39:* 185–189, 1978.

Harosymia, Stefan J., Horne, Marcia D., and Lewis, Sally C. A longitudinal study of disability group acceptance. *Rehab Lit, 37:* 98–102, 1976.

Jones, Reginald L., and Sisk, Dorothy. Early perceptions of orthopedic disability. *Rehab Lit, 31:* 34–38, 1970.

Kvaraceus, William C., and Hayes, E. Nelson. (Eds.). *If Your Child Is Handicapped.* Boston: Porter Sargent, 1969.

Livneh, Hanoch. Disability and monstrosity: Further comments. *Rehab Lit, 41:* 280–283, 1980.

Livneh, Hanoch. On the origins of negative attitudes toward people With disabilities. *Rehab Lit, 43:* 338–347, 1982.

Marenelli, Robert P., and Dell Orto, Arthur E. *The Social Psychological and Social Impact of Physical Disability.* New York: Springer, 1977.

Olshansky, Simon. Stigma: Its meaning and its problems for vocational rehabilitation agencies. *Rehab Lit, 26:* 71–72, 1965.

Ruffner, Robert. Image and identity: Marketing disabled adults in the media. *Disabled USA,* 6 5–7, 1982.

Seethamma, Hampapur N., and Majumder, Ranjitk. New rehabilitation law requires a clearer definition of handicap. In Spiegal, Allen D., Podair, Simon, and Florio, Eunice (Eds.), *Rehabilitating People with Disabilities into the Mainstream of Society.* Park Ridge, NJ: Noyes Medical, 1981.

Thurer, Shari. Disability and monstrosity: A look at literary distortions of handicapped conditions." *Rehab Lit, 41* 12–15, 1980.

Weinberg, Nancy. Social stereotyping the physically handicapped. *Rehab Lit, 23:* 115–124, 1976.

Weinberg, Nancy, and Santana, Rosina. Comic books: Champions of the disabled stereotype. *Rehab Lit, 39:* 327–331, 1978.

Weinberg, Nancy, and Williams, Judy. How the physically disabled perceived their disabilities. *J Rehab, 44:* 31–33, 1978.

Wilson, Donald V. Leprosy and the attitude of society. *Rehab Lit, 31:* 13–15, 1970.

Wright, Beatrice A. *Physical Disability: A Psychological Approach.* New York: Harper & Row, 1960.

Additional Readings

Barker, Roger G. Concepts of disabilities. *Pers Guid J, 43:* 371–374, 1964.

Baskin, B. The handicapped in children's literature. *English Record, 26:* 91–99, 1974.

Byrd, E. Keith, Byrd, P. Dianne, and Allen, Conrad M. Television programming and disability. *J Appl Rehab Couns, 8:* 28–32, 1977.

English, R. William. Combating stigma toward physically disabled persons. *Rehab Res Practice Rev, 2:* 1–17, 1971.

Forgus, Ronald H. *Perception.* New York: McGraw-Hill, 1966.

McDaniel, James W. *Physical Disability and Human Behavior.* New York: Pergamon Press, 1970.

Nelson, Robert. *Creating Community Acceptance for Handicapped People.* Springfield, IL: Charles C Thomas, 1978.

Rickard, Thomas E., Triandis, Harry C., and Patterson, C. H. Indices of employer prejudice toward disabled applicants. *J Appl Psychol, 47:* 52–55, 1963.

Thoreson, Richard W., and Kerr, Barbara A. The stigmatizing aspects of severe disability: Strategies for change. *J Appl Rehab Couns, 9:* 21–25, 1978.

Tuller, N. R. The effects of educational films on attitude change. *Educ Persp, 15:* 22–28, 1976.

Chapter 5

ETHNIC GROUP CHARACTERISTICS

I see myself within the world, against the world, but not really a part of the world.

Donald Petty (1979)

The statement above was made by a person with a disability, but it could easily have been made by a member of an ethnic minority group. In many ways, people with physical disabilities are subjected to discrimination and segregation similar to that which ethnic minorities receive (Barker et al., 1953; Chesler, 1965). Few writers disagree with the statement that ethnic minorities and people with disabilities are marginal to the general population. Ethnic minority adults tend to accept their own children with disabilities. However, this attitude is not characteristic of their children. Stephen Richardson and associates (1944) found that white, black, and Puerto Rican children ranked children without disabilities higher on a social scale than children with disabilities. Daniel Alessi and William Anthony (1969) found that children with disabilities rank persons with disabilities low in social status.

Persons with disabilities and ethnic minorities fit Erving Goffman's (1963) concept of *stigmatized individuals:* "The stigmatized individual finds himself in an arena of detailed argument and discussion concerning what he ought to think of himself. . . . To his other troubles he must add that of being simultaneously pushed in several directions by professionals who tell him what he should do and feel about what he is and isn't" (p. 124). In most instances, stigmatized people internalize a sense of personal devaluation and second-class citizenship. According to Carolyn Vash (1981), this is the primal human fear at the individual level.

SIMILARITIES AND DIFFERENCES

Extreme negative self-devaluation is an important factor in cultural meanings of ethnicity and physical disability. Such devaluation centers on the belief that an individual with a disability does not have the ability to perform tasks that people without a disability take for granted. Extreme self-devaluation can result in (1) loss of emotional stability, (2) loss of sustained personal pleasure, and (3) loss of physical and economic independence. In short, individuals with disabilities become sociopsychologically and economically crippled.

This crippling process is known as *handicapism*. Robert Bogdan and Douglas Biklen (1981) defined *handicapism* as "a set of assumptions and practices that promote the differential and unequal treatment of people because of apparent or assumed physical, mental, or behavioral differences.... Handicapism arises in the contacts between handicapped and so-called typical people as well as in the private conversations of typical people when the handicapped are not present" (pp. 16, 18).

Numerous writers have pointed out that not only attitudinal but also architectural and mobility barriers create social isolation and economic and social dependency in people with disabilities. Like ethnic minorities, these people are plagued by stereotyped beliefs about their greatly limited mental and physical capacities. However, there are differences between the two groups. People with physical disabilities are not a distinct cultural group, whereas ethnic minorities are. People with disabilities often are isolated and must suffer their privations without the support of other persons with similar disabilities. Being a member of an ethnic minority group allows individuals to attribute their deprivations to racism, while people with disabilities tend to personalize their deprivations.

Even the family with a person who has a disability does not automatically share his or her low social status, but it is common for ethnic minority family members all to share the same status. John Gliedman and William Roth (1980) correctly pointed out that disabilities are not produced or transmitted in a way that parallels racial or ethnic characteristics. Most children with physical disabilities have nondisabled parents, and most parents with physical disabilities have children who do not have disabilities.

Comparing Americans with physical disabilities with black Americans during the late 1960s, Leonard Kriegel (1961) draws a poignant analogy: "For the cripple, the black man is a model because he is on intimate terms with a terror that does not recognize his existence and is yet distinctly personal. He is in the process of discovering what he is, and he has known for a long time what society conceives him to be. . . . The assumption about me was simple: I should be grateful for whatever existence I could scrape together" (pp. 416–417). The "place" of blacks and individuals with disabilities has too long been behind able-bodied white Americans.

Another important difference is that people with disabilities are not seen by high-status persons as social and economic threats, but ethnic minorities are. There have never been restrictive covenants preventing people with disabilities from purchasing mortgages, for example, although in some neighborhoods there is considerable community resistance to people with disabilities moving in. Similar to their fear of ethnic minorities, the belief of many people is that people with disabilities will exhibit antisocial behavior and will cause real estate values to go down.

Moreover, while ethnic minorities can take pride in their differences, uniqueness, and histories, people with disabilities have a more difficult time finding reason for pride in their physical impairments. However, as Don Galloway (1981) pointed out, a growing number of them are gaining pride: "The reason that there is disabled pride comes from whatever you've done with what you've got. . . . Disabled can be a positive thing. Being black or disabled can bring an added dimension to the realities of life. . . . Hell, yeah, blindness is beautiful. Not in itself, but we have made it that, a positive thing" (p. 188). Thus, ethnic minorities and people with disabilities are the same in some aspects but different in others.

In retrospect, all groups in the United States are people of considerable cultural diversity. Although all segments of our population share the same physical disabilities and patterns of adjustment, there are recognizable differences in subcultural attitudes, interests, history, and dialects. Furthermore, people with disabilities bring to social settings differences based on masculine and feminine roles, urban and rural backgrounds, ethnic identity, and social class.

MASCULINE AND FEMININE ROLES. Until recently in this nation, males and females were expected to play different roles. One of the first lessons children learned from those around them was that their behavior must accord with that generally considered appropriate to their sex. A boy was not expected to take on feminine characteristics, and a girl was handicapped if she were not feminine in dress, speech, and aspirations. "Good boys" and "good girls" were those who engaged in sex-appropriate behavior.

In their study of women with disabilities, Michelle Fine and Adrienne Asch (1981) concluded that females more than males are handicapped by the economy, society, and their own negative self-images. Females with disabilities are more likely to internalize their handicaps. A black woman with a disability wrote, "Of the three minorities of which I am a member, the handicap has dominated my life" (Fine and Asch, p. 238). One would have to be devoid of sensitivity to misinterpret the following message:

> The first time the doubt that I belonged to this particular planet struck me, was a glorious, calm, blue-skied day when I was twelve years old. Lying flat on my back in the garden, staring at the sky, I was thinking of growing up. Until that moment I think I had somehow believed that when I grew up I would become "normal," i.e. without a disability.... That momentous day I suddenly realized that my life was not going to be like that at all. I was going to be just as I had always been — very small, funnily shaped, unable to walk. It seemed at that moment that the sky cracked. [Campling, 1981, pp. 23–24]

Females with disabilities often grow up believing that they are ugly. Some of them believe they are more like vegetables than people; others feel like imbeciles. Female children with disabilities frequently are not raised as females. Rather, they are raised as asexual persons; they doubt their abilities to menstruate or even have breasts. Consequently, a truncated societal rank order of acceptable persons in descending order is: (1) white males without disabilities, (2) white females without disabilities, (3) nonwhite males without disabilities, (4) nonwhite females without disabilities, (5) white males with disabilities, (6) nonwhite males with disabilities, (7) white females with disabilities, and (8) nonwhite females with disabilities.

RURAL AND URBAN BACKGROUNDS. Although they are not as striking as they used to be, differences in language, attitudes, and interests between rural and urban disabled people still exist. However, ethnic identity and social class rather than place of origin mainly determine the social orientation of a person with a disability.

ETHNIC IDENTITY. Most Americans can trace their ancestry back to some country across the oceans. Each ethnic group has enriched this culture with its own particular types of music, food, customs, and dress. It usually takes two or more generations for the members of a new immigrant group to become absorbed into the life of the community sufficiently that they lose their separate identity. Some ethnic groups, mainly those of dark skin colors, never achieve total assimilation. Moreover, as seen in Chapter 3, it is almost impossible for individuals with physical disabilities to climb in the pot and melt away.

SOCIAL CLASSES. The United States has rather clearly defined social classes, and people with physical disabilities tend to number disproportionately in the lower classes. Equal employment opportunity laws and programs of the past two decades have resulted in a substantial increase in the number of gainfully employed ethnic minorities, but they have done little to improve conditions for ethnic minority workers with disabilities.

BLACK AMERICANS

Black children with disabilities begin life facing higher survival odds than their white peers. They are more likely to die in infancy than white babies. If a black baby lives, the chance of losing his or her mother in childbirth is four times as high as that of the white baby. The black baby usually is born into a family that lives in the inner city. (Over 60 percent of the black American population does.) The family is larger than its white counterpart, and it is likely to be crowded into dilapidated housing—quarters structurally unsound or unable to keep out cold, rain, snow, rats, or pests (Henderson, 1979).

With more mouths to feed, more babies to clothe, and more needs to satisfy, the black family is forced to exist on a median family income that is barely half the median white family income. When black children with disabilities go to school, they usually find it no avenue to adequate living, much less to fame or fortune. Further, because black children generally are taught in slum schools, with inferior teachers, equipment, and facilities, the educational gap between blacks with disabilities and whites with disabilities, of the same age, often approaches three or four years.

In most communities heavily populated by black Americans, low- and middle-income groups live in extremely close proximity. This situation is not primarily caused by a "natural selection" process but rather by *de facto* housing segregation. Consequently, the plight of poverty-stricken black Americans is distorted if only census tract data are examined. Black "haves" appear less affluent, and black "have-nots" seem less disadvantaged than they actually are. There is, in short, a much wider gap between the black middle and lower classes than is statistically apparent. Both groups closely approximate their white counterparts in income and living styles. Black Americans with disabilities, however, are a minority within a minority.

Black Americans are the most difficult ethnic group to categorize. The difficulty stems mainly from slavery, in which African heritages were almost entirely lost through assimilation with non-African cultures. Even so, the following generalizations typify traditional African American cultural conditioning.

EXTENDED FAMILY. The black family is sometimes extended bilaterally, but often it is maternally oriented. The black extended family is a closely knit group, frequently consisting of grandparents, aunts, uncles, nieces, nephews, and cousins. Roles are interchanged within the black family more frequently than in most nonblack families. This sharing of decisions and jobs in the home stabilizes the family during crises situations. Family members with disabilities are cared for by all persons in the home.

KINSHIP BONDS. Children with physical disabilities are loved. Disability refers to luck; it has little to do with black children being accepted. Besides, all children, able-bodied and disabled, are proof of an individual's manhood or womanhood, and caring for them is proof of the person's humanity. Generally, when blacks with disabilities marry or otherwise reach adulthood, they live with their parents or settle close to them or other relatives. Family unity, loyalty, and cooperation are part of the black life-style. (These values also are strongly held by the other ethnic groups discussed in this chapter.)

AUTHORITY AND DISCIPLINE. Childhood in the black community revolves around assertive behavior and challenging authority. There is a constant crossing of wills. Through this process children with disabilities learn the acceptable limits of their behavior. Discipline tends to be harsh, strict, and preoccupied with teaching children respect for their elders, respect for authority, responsibility for themselves, and an understanding of what it means to be black and disabled in America. Brenda Clark (1981) described this conditioning: "I don't think I was overprotected or put aside. I feel that I was able to do just as much as my sisters and brothers and just as much as my friends. If I wanted to survive and be like everybody else I had to prove that I could do all the things that able-bodied people were able to do" (p. 131).

RELIGIOUS ORIENTATION. As a whole, black Americans are highly religious. Most of them are Protestant. The church offers much-needed spiritual hope to disabled persons who live in oppressive environments. The church also offers reasons for accepting individuals with disabilities.

ACHIEVEMENT AND WORK ORIENTATIONS. Contrary to popular notion, most black parents pass on to their children high achievement aspirations. However, many black homes lack middle-class role models for children to emulate. The desire to achieve has forced many black families to internalize a strong work orientation that makes palatable the unskilled and semiskilled jobs available in the discriminatory job markets within which most persons with disabilities work.

FOLK MEDICINE. African health practices make little distinction between physicians and nurses; both attend to the physical, emotional, and spiritual health of the patient. According to traditional African beliefs, both living and dead things influence an individual's health. In addition, health is directly related to nature. To be in harmony with nature is to have good health, whereas illness reflects being out of harmony with nature. It is common for parents to treat their children's disabilities with home remedies.

MEXICAN AMERICANS

Disabled Mexican Americans reflect a variety of cultural patterns that are influenced by their parental heritage and the length of time their families have been American citizens. Second– and third-generation descendents of agricultural workers tend to be poor. A third group is formed by the first-generation children of *braceros,* farm workers who have recently migrated from Mexico. The first two groups are likely to be Americanized: They have little knowledge of their Spanish heritage, and they speak little or no Spanish. Children of migrant workers speak fluent Spanish and hold tightly to Mexican customs and traditions. All Spanish groups are discriminated against by the Anglos, the white American majority. Julian Samora (1966) noted that in some communities Mexican Americans are the victims of more discrimination and segregation than black Americans.

Census projections indicate that the total Hispanic American population may soon exceed the black American population. In addition to Mexicans and Puerto Ricans, a sizable number of legal and illegal immigrants come from Argentina, Peru, and Venezuela. Part of the difficulty in accurately counting and classifying Hispanic immigrants is due to the tendency of non–Puerto Rican Hispanics to list themselves as Puerto Rican in order to gain full rights as American citizens. In Texas and California it is estimated that 1 million illegal immigrants have entered from Mexico. Their *barrios* (communities) tend to reflect the same economic and physical conditions as black neighborhoods.

In many ways Mexican Americans epitomize both racial integration and cultural separatism. This duality is clearly seen in a brief review of Mexican history. The Aztecs were intermarried with their Spanish conquerors and with Indian tribes hostile to the Aztecs. The children of these mixed marriages were called *mestizos. Criollos,* pure-blooded Spanish people born in Mexico, largely disappeared through intermarriage. Blacks from Africa, brought into Mexico during the colonial period as slaves, married Indians, and their offspring were called *zambos. Zambos* and *mestizos* later intermarried, causing the so-called Negro blood to disappear.

Although they are a racially mixed people, the heritage of Mexican Americans is quite similar. Some Mexican Americans prefer to be called *Chicanos.* Others prefer *Latino,* and still others prefer *Hispanic.* The word *Chicano* stems from the Mexican Indian Nahuatl word *Mechicano.* The first syllable is dropped, and *Chicano* is left. It is an old term for the American of Mexican descent. The Chicano movement (or *Chicanismo*) represents a commitment to the improvement of life for all Spanish-speaking Americans and Americans of Mexican descent.

Programs that work well for Mexican Americans with disabilities may not work well for other Latino persons with disabilities because of subcultural differences. For example, knowing that a person speaks Spanish may be inadequate cultural knowledge. There are qualitative differences between the language of Latinos who are monolingual Spanish and that of Latinos who are bilingual Spanish-English. Furthermore, Spanish has many dialects — those brought to the United States by Latino immigrants and several that have developed in this country. A discussion of some of the common characteristics of Mexican Americans follows.

LA RAZA (THE RACE). All Latin Americans are united by cultural and spiritual bonds believed to have emanated from God. Because God controls all events, Mexican Americans tend to be more present oriented than future oriented. The influence of the Roman Catholic church on *la Raza* is pervasive: Mexican Americans are born into, get married, work, die, and are buried under the auspices of religious ceremonies. A disability is likely to be viewed as God's will.

FAMILY LOYALTY. The familial role is the most important, and the family is the second most cherished institution in Mexican American society. The worst sin is to violate one's obligations to the church; next comes the family. Family members with disabilities are loved and protected.

RESPECT. The oldest man in the household is the family leader. Respect is accorded on the basis of age and sex. The old are given more respect than the young, and men receive more respect than women. Latino families are based on family solidarity and male superiority.

MACHISMO. All Hispanic cultures prescribe that men are stronger, more reliable, and more intelligent than women. *Machismo* dictates that males show a high degree of individuality outside the family. Weakness in male behavior is looked down on. Consequently, Mexican American males with disabilities often try to hide their physical disabilities so as not to appear weak.

COMPADRAZGO. The Mexican American family is extended by the institution of *compadrazgo,* a special ceremonial bond between a child's parents and godparents. Often the bond between *compadres* is as strong as that between brothers and sisters.

FOLK MEDICINE. Humoral pathology is an important aspect of Latin American and Spanish folk medicine. Their simplified form of Greek humoral pathology was elaborated in the Arab world, brought to Spain as scientific medicine during the period of Moslem domination, and transmitted to America at the time of the Spanish Conquest. According to humoral medical beliefs, the basic functions of the body are regulated by four bodily fluids, or "humors," each of which is characterized by a combination of heat or cold with wetness or dryness. Disabilities are treated with hot and cold home remedies.

PUERTO RICANS

Puerto Rico is an island in the Caribbean approximately 1,000 miles from Miami and 1,600 miles from New York. Puerto Rico's population of almost 4 million represents a density greater than that of China, India, or Japan. As a result of the Jones Act of 1917, all Puerto Ricans are American citizens. The island population is a mixture of Taino Indians, Africans, and Spaniards. Puerto Rican skin colors range from white to black, with shades and mixtures in between (Maldonado-Denis, 1972).

Mainland American–raised Puerto Ricans are sometimes called Neo-Ricans. Neo-Ricans are mainly English speakers; few speak fluent Spanish. Despite dissimilar backgrounds, Puerto Ricans tend to be labeled *black* and subjected to the same prejudices inflicted on Black Americans. Although many Puerto Ricans are reluctant to adopt American life-styles, the following characteristics typify Puerto Rican culture.

SENSE OF DIGNITY. *Respecto* demands that proper attention be given to culturally prescribed rituals such as shaking hands and standing up to greet and say good-bye to people. A sense of dignity is present in all important interpersonal relationships. There is also dignity in the way individuals live with their disabilities.

PERSONALISMO. Personal contact is established by Puerto Ricans before beginning a business relationship. It is important to exchange personal life data (such as size of family and family members' names and ages) before talking business or about one's disability.

INDIVIDUALISM. Puerto Ricans place high value on safeguarding against group pressure to violate an individual's integrity. This makes it difficult for disabled Puerto Ricans to accept the concept of *teamwork* or to relinquish their individuality to conform to a rehabilitation regimen. Lack of conformity reduces the importance of the Roman Catholic Church in the lives of Puerto Ricans, most of whom are Catholic.

CLEANLINESS. Great emphasis is placed on being clean and well dressed. To Puerto Ricans, looking good includes wearing bright colors and, frequently, styles rich in ornament.

FEAR OF AGGRESSION. Puerto Rican children are discouraged from fighting, even in self-defense. A Puerto Rican idiom describes this conditioning: *Juego do mano, juego de villano.* ("Pushing and shoving, even in play, makes one a villain.") Survival in urban slum neighborhoods forces many Puerto Rican children to be villains, especially when defending their siblings and friends who have disabilities.

COMPADRAZGO AND MACHISMO. *Compadrazgo* and *machismo* are operative in Puerto Rican culture in the same manner as in Mexican American culture. Like blacks and Mexicans, Puerto Ricans love children, and disabilities are neither frowned on nor ridiculed.

FOLK MEDICINE. For a discussion of Puerto Rican folk medicine, *see* the section pertaining to Mexican Americans. The two cultures are quite similar in this respect.

AMERICAN INDIANS

There are approximately 300 Indian tribes in the United States. Some are bilingual, and others are not, nor is there a common tribal language. That is why sign language became the chief means of intertribal communication. Currently, American Indians and Alaskan Natives are at the bottom of the economic ladder in the United States. They have the highest rates of unemployment and school dropouts, live in the most dilapidated housing, and in some parts of the country are accorded the lowest social status. These conditions reflect both what white Americans have done to the Indians and what Indians have not been able to do for themselves (Deloria, Jr., 1973).

Finally realizing that this situation is not an Indian problem but rather an American problem, the federal government has begun to phase out government-controlled Indian bureaus, reservations, and assistance programs, including schools, hospitals, and clinics. Each of these short-sighted solutions has in the past contributed to the psychological emasculation of Indian men, the demoralization of Indian women, and the alienation of Indian children. In other words, as a whole, government programs have failed to assist Indians in their efforts to maintain individual dignity and cultural identity while achieving success in the larger society.

Most of the disabled Native American population lives on 40 million acres of reservation in thirty states. Part of their plight is revealed in the following statistics: Indians have 100 million fewer acres of land today than in 1887. Their average life expectancy is forty-five years. Nearly 60 percent of the adult Indian population has less than an eighth-grade education. Infant mortality is more than 10 percent above the national average. The majority of Native American families have annual incomes below $6,000; 75 percent have annual incomes below $5,000. Indian unemployment is almost ten times the national average.

Conflicts between white and Indian cultures are found on reservations, in small towns, and in big cities. The strain shows up in many ways, including juvenile delinquency, adult crime, and alcoholism. Historically, non-Indians have looked at Indian tribes but have failed to see the deplorable social, psychological, and physical deprivations. Some non-Indians tend to think that because one exceptional disabled Indian has managed to succeed, others should be able to do so without much assistance. Generally, the following characteristics apply to traditional American Indians.

PRESENT ORIENTED. Indians are taught to live in the present and not to be concerned about what tomorrow will bring. Non-Indians tend to be future oriented; they are constantly destroying the past and building the future.

TIME CONSCIOUSNESS. Many earlier Indian tribes had no word for *time*. Thus, historically, the emphasis was placed on doing as opposed to going to do something or being punctual. Unlike non-Indians who rush to meetings to be punctual, Indians try to finish current activities. Most persons with disabilities, Indian and non-Indian, develop this same concept of time: "Generally we are not usually concerned with time per se, but rather with its utilization. . . . Common functions such as getting dressed, preparing a meal, or other tasks that are taken for granted by the non-disabled, may occupy a place of major importance to an individual with disability. Time is finite and if daily living requirements involve longer time frames, a person's choices of activities become restricted" (Vacc and Clifford, 1980, p. 248).

GIVING. The Indian who gives the most to others is respected. In many tribes, saving money or accumulating consumer goods results in ostracism. Helping individuals with disabilities is part of this ethic.

RESPECT FOR AGE. Like the other ethnic groups discussed in this chapter, the Indian increases the respect accorded an individual according to his or her age. Indian leadership is seldom given to the young.

COOPERATION. Indians place great value on working together and sharing resources. Failure to achieve a personal goal is believed to be the result of competition. Persons with disabilities are encouraged to contribute to family and tribal activities.

HARMONY WITH NATURE. The Indian believes in living in harmony with nature. He or she accepts the world as it is and does not try to destroy it. Along with this belief goes a belief in taking from the environment only what is needed to live.

EXTENDED FAMILY. The American Indian family network is radically different from other extended family units in the United States. The typical non-Indian extended family includes three generations within a single household. American Indian families include several households representing relatives along both vertical and horizontal lines. Grandparents are official and symbolic family leaders. In addition, namesakes (formalized through a religious ceremony) become the same as parents in the family network.

FOLK MEDICINE. The Indian medicine man is a vivid reminder that long before physicians, nurses, social workers, and counselors intruded into their lives, Native Americans had folk cures for physical and mental disabilities. Upon reflection, it is no more illogical to believe in spirits that cannot be seen than in germs that cannot be seen. An example of Indian folk medicine is seen in traditional Navajo culture, which asserts that illness is a sign that a person is out of harmony with nature. Indian religion and medicine are virtually indistinguishable. Medicine men, singing, rituals, and chants are important aspects of treatment for illness.

ASIAN AMERICANS

The plight of poverty-stricken disabled Asian Americans is vividly captured in Los Angeles and San Francisco Chinatown statistics: More than one-third of the Chinatown families are poverty stricken; three-fourths of all housing units are substandard; rents have tripled in the past five years; more than half the adults have only a grade-school education; juvenile delinquency is increasing; the suicide rate is three times the national average. Stanley Sue and Derald Sue (1973) cautioned that most Asian Americans are neither poverty stricken nor poorly educated. Many of the following values that characterize traditional Chinese are applicable to most traditional Asian cultures.

FILIAL PIETY. There is unquestioning respect for and deference to authority. Above all else, there is the expectation that each individual will comply with familial and social authority.

PARENT-CHILD RELATIONSHIP. Children defer to their parents, especially in communication, which is one-way from parents to children.

SELF-CONTROL. Strong negative feelings are seldom verbalized. Assertive and individualistic people are considered crude and poorly socialized.

FATALISM. Resignation and pragmatism characterize the manner in which Chinese Americans deal with change in nature and social settings.

SOCIAL MILIEU. Chinese Americans are other-directed, and therefore they are greatly concerned with how their significant others view and react to them. Social solidarity is highly valued.

INCONSPICUOUSNESS. Taught to avoid calling attention to themselves, Chinese Americans are likely to be silent in public settings. This is especially true of Chinese with disabilities.

SHAME AND GUILT. Since Chinese Americans are taught to respect authority and maintain filial piety toward their parents and their ancestors, a violation of this cultural norm results in feelings of shame and guilt. The Chinese family is a continuum from past to future whose membership includes not only the present generation but also the dead and the unborn.

FOLK MEDICINE. Asian folk medicine and philosophies have a strong Chinese influence. This is the result of early Chinese migration throughout Asia. Comparing Chinese, Japanese, Filipino, and Korean medicine shows that similarity. All four have similar philosophies concerning nutrition, acupuncture, and herbology. The art and science of Chinese medicine goes back at least 5,000 years. Unlike Western medicine, which emphasizes disease and cure, Asian medicine focuses on prevention. Even so, considerable attention is given to correcting disabilities and relieving pain.

The theoretical and philosophical foundation of Chinese medicine is the Taoist religion, which seeks a balance in all things. From a Taoist perspective, humans are microcosms within a macrocosm. Human energy of the microcosm interrelates with the universe. Both energy (*Chi*) and sexual energy (*Jing*) are vital life energies. Chi and Jing are kept in balance by Yin and Yang. Yin is feminine, negative, dark, and cold, whereas Yang is masculine, positive, light, and warm. According to Chinese medicine, an imbalance in energy is caused by an improper diet or a strong emotional feeling. Balance or good health may be achieved through the use of appropriate herbs.

LOWER-CLASS ETHNIC MINORITIES

Some helpers fail to realize that lower-class ethnic minorities with disabilities are people who have feelings similar to their own. Most lower-class people are sensitive, concerned, and easily embarrassed. An old proverb states, "Poverty [or disability] does not destroy virtue, nor does wealth bestow it." Oblivious to this fact, too many middle-class helpers respond to lower-class people in patronizing and humiliating ways. When professional helpers consider themselves the experts, they usually rule out a peer relationship with lower-class people, especially lower-class people with disabilities.

Before any helper, professional or nonprofessional, can optimally interact with disabled lower-class people, he or she must be aware of the physical and social environment characterizing low-income communities. This includes an awareness of what lower-class homes are like. More than anything else, it is necessary to understand the basic factors of survival within subcultures of urban poverty, for that is where most lower-class people with disabilities spend their time.

Physical Environment

Physical appearance is one of the most revealing characteristics of a low-income neighborhood. Neglect and disorder are common. Public services—sanitation inspections and garbage collection—often appear to be nonexistent. Buildings are in advanced states of deterioration, highlighting structual neglect and social decline. Slum neighborhoods are overcrowded with buildings, and the buildings are overcrowded with people. The population consists mainly of people who are not welcome in other areas or who cannot afford to live elsewhere. Infant and maternal mortality rates are high; so, too, are unemployment and underemployment. Vice is rampant in the slums, although it is by no means confined to this area. Furthermore, slums are the habitat of marginal people and the hiding place for fugitives.

A low-income community can be thought of as an area of anonymity and alienation. Except for a few families that do not have the means to move, most of the population is transient, moving from one low-income neighborhood to another. The slums gradually acquire a character clearly different from that of other areas of the community. In many ways, city slums are ports of entry for rural migrants and points of departure for the upwardly mobile. As each city grows, it creates a belt of bleak, barren, soot-covered, physically deteriorated structures around its core.

Home and School Environments

Considering the kind of community they live in makes it easy to see the special problems lower-class people with disabilities face. Adequate recreational facilities are almost nonexistent, and therefore disabled children play in the streets and alleys. Parents usually must work long hours to earn barely enough for minimal subsistence. When at home, lower-class parents often are tired and worrying about where the next meal will come from or how they are going to pay next month's rent. They seldom listen or pay attention to their children. This is not to say that their children are neglected and unloved but instead that they often *feel* neglected and unloved. Parental frustration tolerance levels are low, and lower-class parents tend to discipline their children with a "good whipping." There are not usually any books in the home. If books are present, lighting may be so inadequate that it is difficult for children to read, if they know how.

A large number of lower-class children have chronic skin infections, dental problems, and chronically infected ears that can lead to deafness. Greatly restricted diets further reduce lower-class mothers' chances of giving birth to well babies. Thus, physical infirmities are commonplace.

Some lower-class parents believe that it is more important for their children to get out and work than to continue their education. Thus, many children are encouraged to leave school and get a job before graduating from high school. Sometimes children must work after school in order for their families to have enough money to live. Children with disabilities frequently feel guilty for not being able to "pull their own weight" by working.

Most of the poor are not recipients of welfare. The typical lower-class parents have less than an eighth-grade education; if employed, they are employed as unskilled and semiskilled workers. The family's income per person often is considerably less than the minimum wage. These people do not get their names in the news as outstanding representatives of their ethnic group, nor do they show up very often as criminals in crime statistics. On the one hand, their children manage to keep out of trouble and are not what might generally be called uneducable. On the other hand, their children are likely to be overlooked when teachers are recommending someone to pose for a picture or to represent the school. This is especially true of ethnic minority children with physical disabilities.

For discussion purposes, lower-class children with disabilities can be divided into three groups. The first is the children whose families lack substantial material wealth but who receive enough warmth and emotional support from their parents to assure normal school development. This encompasses the majority of poor children. The second type of children lack both material and parental support; their parents are indifferent to their needs, largely through ignorance. With proper care, these children can make a satisfactory school adjustment. The children in the third group come from families in which the parents are mentally retarded or psychotic. Family life for these children is characterized by filth, inadequate diet, and extreme alienation. Consequently, they are psychologically and organically fragile persons, easily bruised or broken. They are truly disadvantaged.

Lower-class children with disabilities are in a narrowly constructed psychological box, built for them by their parents and community, from which they can seldom escape. Behaving as anyone would in such a box, they become hostile toward adults who constantly demand a higher degree of restraint and self-control than they exhibit themselves, hostile toward teachers who clutter the box with unsolicited facts, assignments, and rules, and hostile toward themselves for being disabled. Most lower-class parents sense these feelings and try unsuccessfully to help their children out of the box, but, alas, school and home forces shut the psychological box with the children still inside.

ESTABLISHING TRUST

The initial step for nondisabled people who want to help ethnic minorities with disabilities is to build trust. The communication of trust must first come from the would-be helpers, who should use verbal and nonverbal signs of acceptance and respect. Hostility-producing words and phrases such as *crip* and *you people* should be avoided. An initial assessment must be made as to how a person prefers to be addressed. In formal settings, most young persons with disabilities prefer to be addressed by their first names, whereas most older persons with disabilities prefer to be addressed by "Doctor," "Miss," "Mrs.," or "Mr." and their last names.

Nonverbal interactions that may be construed to mean non-acceptance include refusal to sit down when making a home visit, reluctance to shake hands with persons with disabilities, physically moving away from them, and making facial expressions that imply disgust. Some ethnic minorities consider it bad manners to stare at others. Therefore, helpers should not be surprised if individuals with disabilities do not look at them when talking.

When a person with a disability exhibits paranoid responses or hostile behavior, a sensitive helper will recognize these as possible adaptive mechanisms that the individual uses to survive in his or her everyday world. It is important for helpers to accept each disabled person where he or she is and implement an effective means of communication. Studies of people who are effective communicating with those with physical disabilities suggest that, like Abraham H. Maslow's self-actualized people, they have few ego-centered thoughts during the interaction. Their attention is focused on the disabled persons. Methodologically, their major effort centers on collecting and correctly understanding data. The first rule of communication is to understand the other person's value system. This implies respect for different ethnic-group values.

Most helpers walk a thin line, which they fall off from time to time. They must care, but not too much, or they will lose their objectivity. The task is formidable: Clients must be given the best chance of social adjustment and the least chance of disillusionment. This of course, is the perennial problem of humanely managing emotions and realistically maximizing client abilities. Clearly, considerable human relations skill is needed to perform these delicate tasks. In this imperfect world, persons with disabilities expect much from the individuals to whom they entrust their lives and aspirations.

The helping relationship is necessarily based on acceptance, expectation, support, and stimulation. *Acceptance* means unconditionally giving oneself to and receiving another person. The individual accepting an ethnic minority group person is communicating: "I will apply my human relations skills to help you. As I do this, I will try to meet your needs, to understand you and to respect your right to retain your own ethnic identity." In most instances, these nurturing qualities are not easily taught or freely applied. Yet, the ability to accept an individual's ethnicity is the *sine qua non* of the helping relationship.

Expectation means the projection that responsive behavior will occur. Helpers expect those being helped to be cooperative, while those being helped expect their helpers to assist in devising the best possible rehabilitation plan for them. Usually, professional helpers are quite explicit and direct in their expectations, but ethnic minority clients with disabilities tend to be less direct and to rely more on nonverbal behavior to express themselves.

For some helpers the support and stimulus needed to continue working with persons with disabilities comes from successful actions. For others it comes from the belief that their interventions, even when unsuccessful, are needed. People with disabilities, on the other hand, receive their support and stimulus largely from satisfactory social adjustment. The more effective helpers are able to project to ethnic minority people their genuine concern, empathy, and technical skills. However, even these attributes may not be sufficient to dissolve an ethnic minority individual's fears and anxieties. There is something inherently disconcerting about having to seek help.

Although talking may not allay fears and anxieties, it can certainly pave the way for this to occur. It is not usual for clients to remain silent or inarticulate or to talk about unrelated issues. As clients tell their needs, glibly or haltingly, helpers should communicate that they not only understand but also empathize. Failure to do this will result in the termination of the relationship. Ethnic minority clients frequently take their cues from helpers. Insensitivity to an individual's beliefs and fears may result in the premature termination of the interaction. Most persons with disabilities need time to talk, to listen, and to learn new behavior options.

When needs are expressed and accepted, the distance between person being helped and helper is spanned. As the relationship unfolds, the special background of the helper comes to the center of the interaction. Both verbally and nonverbally, an effective helper will communicate acceptance. When ethnic minority persons with disabilities are nourished and sustained by contact with caring persons, the relationship is not only good but also helpful. All helpers would do well to remember that most people are like the philosopher in James Stephens's *The Crock of Gold* (1946), who said, "I have learned that the head does not hear anything until the heart has listened, and that what the heart knows today the head will understand tomorrow" (p. 128).

SUMMARY

The authors do not want to delude anyone into thinking that it is an easy task to establish trust and rapport with ethnic minorities who have disabilities. It is not. No group has been subjected to as much suffering at the hands of society as ethnic minorities. They may be described, borrowing a phrase from Martin Luther King, Jr., as victims of creative brutality. Moreover, the plight of people with disabilities should not be attributed solely to the able-bodied; much of it has grown out of inhuman technology and short-sighted government regulations. Many of the so-called handicapped programs designed to help people with disabilities merely increase unemployment and welfare rolls while simultaneously killing individual initiative and self-determination.

Nor does trust come easy from people who do not trust themselves. Too many ethnic minorities with disabilities have lost faith in themselves. They learn to suffer quietly. Religion tends to make this a less difficult process; "Nobody knows the trouble I've seen," begins a Negro spiritual. Perhaps their general faith in God and particular faith in a religion offer rays of hope to these people:

When everything seems lost, praying just seems to make things less hopeless. Almost all religions teach obedience to their doctrines, to authority, to parents, but seldom to one's own inner feelings.

W. E. B. Dubois (1961) was writing about black people, but his message is especially relevant to individuals who would intervene in the lives of other ethnic minorities:

> Teach thinkers to think,—a needed knowledge in a day of loose and careless logic; they whose lot is gravest must have the carefulest training to think aright.... Teach the workers to work and the thinkers to think; make carpenters of carpenters, and philosophers of philosophers, and fops of fools. Nor can we pause here. We are training not isolated men but a living group of men,—nay, a group within a group. And the final product of our training must be neither a psychologist nor a brickmason, but a man. And to make men, we must have ideals, broad, pure, and inspiring ends of living. [P. 72]

NOTE TO HELPERS

Professional helpers must go beyond giving lip service to valuing cultural and physical differences. They must take an active stance in protecting these differences. For clients with disabilities, advocacy is a proactive process of empathy and listening rather than telling, supporting the goals identified by persons with disabilities and recognizing when to collaborate with other persons. Helpers can best serve themselves and their clients when they recognize and prepare for conflict situations. Conflict is inevitable in society, but it does not have to be a destructive force that breeds hostility and alienation. Properly channeled, conflict can lead to constructive problem solving.

Both helpers and their clients should understand that social change requires risk taking. However, persons who risk nothing *or everything* are seldom successful. Risking something specific in a thoughtful, calculated manner is the most prudent way to proceed. It is hazardous enough to risk employment and educational opportunities with one's eyes open; to do so in ignorance is to invite needless failure. Although physical disabilities complicate human interactions, they are not irreversible assets or liabilities. The key is what one does with a disability.

While written for professionals who provide counseling/therapy for females, the principles adopted in 1979 by the American Psychological Association's Division of Counseling Psychology are relevant to all helpers working with ethnic minorities and persons with disabilities. The authors have paraphrased the principles below to fit ethnic minorities and persons with disabilities:

1. Professional helpers must be knowledgeable about ethnic minorities and physical differences, particularly with regard to historical, psychological, and social issues.

2. Professional helpers must be aware that assumptions and precepts of theories relevant to their practice may apply differently to ethnic minorities and persons with disabilities. Professional helpers must be aware of the theories that prescribe or limit the potential of ethnic minorities and persons with disabilities.

3. After formal training, professional helpers must continue throughout their professional careers to explore and learn of issues related to ethnic minorities and persons with disabilities.

4. Professional helpers must recognize and be aware of various forms of oppression and how these interact with racism and handicapism.

5. Professional helpers must be knowledgeable and aware of verbal and nonverbal process variables (particularly with regard to power in the helping relationship) as these affect ethnic minorities and persons with disabilities in the helping relationship, so that helper-client interactions are not adversely affected. The need for shared responsibility between clients and helpers must be acknowledged and implemented.

6. Professional helpers must be capable of utilizing skills that are particularly facilitative to ethnic minorities and persons with disabilities in general and specific clients in particular.

7. Professional helpers must ascribe to no preconceived limitations on the direction or nature of the life goals of ethnic minorities and persons with disabilities.

8. Professional helpers must be sensitive to circumstances in which it is more desirable for an ethnic minority or person with a disability to be seen by a helper who is an ethnic minority or a person with a disability.

9. Professional helpers must use nonracist and other non-

demeaning language in counseling/therapy, supervision, teaching, and publications.

10. Professional helpers must not engage in sexual activity with their clients.

11. Professional helpers must be aware of and continually review their own values and biases and the effect of these on their clients.

12. Professional helpers must be aware of how their personal functioning may influence their effectiveness in working with ethnic minorities and persons with disabilities. They must monitor their functioning through consultation, supervision, or therapy, so that it does not adversely affect their work with ethnic minorities and persons with disabilities.

13. Professional helpers must support the elimination of racism and handicapism within institutions and individuals.

REFERENCES

Alessi, D. F. and Anthony, W. A. The uniformity of children's attitudes toward disabilities. *Except Child, 35:* 543–545, 1969.

Barker, R. C., Wright, B. A., Meyerson, L., and Gonick, M. K. *Adjustment to Physical Handicap and Illness: A Survey of the Social Psychology of Physique.* New York: Social Science Research Council, 1953.

Bogdan, Robert, and Biklen, Douglas. handicapism. In Spiegel, Allen D., Podair, Simon, and Fiorito, Eunice (Eds.). *Rehabilitating People with Disabilities into the Mainstream of Society.* Park Ridge, NJ: Noyes Medical, 1981.

Campling, Jo (Ed.). *Images of Ourselves: Women with Disabilities Talking.* Boston: Routledge and Kegan Paul, 1981.

Chesler, M. A. Ethnocentusm and attitudes toward the physically disabled. *Pers Soc Res,* 2:877–882, 1965.

Clark, Brenda. Quoted in Roth, William. *The Handicapped Speak.* Jefferson, NC: McFarland, 1981.

Deloria, Vine, Jr. *God Is Red.* New York: Grosset and Dunlap, 1973.

DuBois, W. E. B. *The Souls of Black Folk.* New York: Fawcett, 1961.

Fine, Michelle, and Asch, Adrienne. Disabled women: Sexism without the pedestal. *Sociol Welfare,* 8:233–248, 1981.

Galloway, Don. Quoted in Roth, William. *The Handicapped Speak.* Jefferson, NC: McFarland, 1981.

Gliedman, John, and Roth, William. *The Unexpected Minority: Handicapped Children in America.* New York: Harcourt Brace Jovanovich, 1980.

Goffman, Erving. *Stigma: Notes on the Management of Spoiled Identity.* Englewood Cliffs, NJ: Prentice-Hall, 1963.

Henderson, George (Ed.). *Understanding and Counseling Ethnic Minorities.* Springfield, IL: Charles C Thomas, 1979.

Kriegel, Leonard. Uncle Tom and Tiny Tim: Some reflections on the cripple as Negro. *Am Scholar, 38*:412–430, 1961.

Maldoldo-Denis, Manuel. *Puerto Rico: A Socio-historic Interpretation.* New York: Random House, 1972.

Petty, Don. What is it like to be deaf-blind? *Consumers Contemporary, 1:* 10–11, 1979.

Richardson, S. A., Hastorf, A. H., Goodman, N., and Dornbusch, S. M. Cultural uniformity in reaction to disabilities. *Am Soc Rev, 26*:241–247, 1961.

Samora, Julian (Ed.). *La Raza: Forgotten Americans.* South Bend, IN: University of Notre Dame Press, 1966.

Stephens, James. *The Crock of Gold.* New York: Macmillan, 1946.

Sue, Stanley, and Sue, Derald. Understanding Asian-Americans: A neglected minority. *Pers Guid J, 5:* 387–389, 1973.

Vacc, Nicholas A., and Clifford, Kerry F. Persons with a disability. In Vacc, Nicholas A., and Wittmer, Joseph P. (Eds.). *Let Me Be Me: Special Populations and the Helping Professional.* Muncie, IN: Accelerated Development, 1980.

Vash, Carolyn. *The Psychology of Disability.* New York: Springer, 1981.

Additional Readings

Albrecht, Gary (Ed.). *The Sociology of Physical Disability and Rehabilitation.* Pittsburgh: University of Pittsburgh Press, 1976.

Cabrera, J. Arturo. *Emerging Faces of the Mexican Americans.* New York: Wm C. Brown, 1971.

Fantini, Mario D., and Cardenas, Rene (Eds.). *Parenting in a Multicultural Society.* Columbus, OH: Charles E. Merrill, 1979.

Felker, Donald W. *Building Positive Self-Concepts.* Minneapolis: Burgess, 1974.

McDaniel, James. *Physical Disability and Human Behavior.* New York: Pergamon Press, 1969.

McGuire, William J., McGuire, Clair V., Child, Pamela, and Fryeoka, Jerry. Salience of ethnicity in the spontaneous self-concept as a function of one's ethnic distinctiveness in the social environment. *J Pers Soc Psychol, 36:* 511–520, 1978.

Smith, William D., Burlew, Ann K., Mosley, Myrtis H., and Whitney, W. Monty. *Minority Issues in Mental Health.* Reading, MA: Addison-Wesley, 1978.

Taylor, Ronald L. Psychosocial development among black children and youth: A re-examination. *Am J Orthopsychiatry, 46:* 4–19, 1976.

Verma, Gajendra, and Bagley, Christopher (Eds.). *Self-Concept, Achievement and Multicultural Educations.* London: Macmillan Press, 1982.

Chapter 6

COPING STYLES

People with disabilities have as many social selves as there are distinct groups of people whose opinion they value. It is extremely painful for them to be rejected by individuals about whom they care. This is a normal reaction. Continued rejection may cause an individual to stop seeking recognition or to change reference groups. Cynical persons are created out of a series of rejections and put-downs. This condition suggests a centrality in which persons with disabilities who receive recognition conform to the peer norms or standards of persons without disabilities. These conformists also are likely to be individuals with disabilities who have high status within their communities. They are not treated the same as the masses of people with disabilities. Thus, differentiation of social status usually results in differentiation of conformity to group norms. Most people with physical disabilities are able to fit into majority group social and economic settings. Unfortunately, too few are allowed to do so; instead, they tend to be relegated to low social status and low-paying jobs.

Rather than focusing on individual needs, most people treat individuals with disabilities as an aggregate. As a whole, parents of children with disabilities are not much different. Instead of encouraging their children to assume responsibility for their own learning and personal growth, many parents cause them to be docile and dependent. Educators contribute to this process, too. Instead of helping these students to optimize their intellectual abilities, most teachers tend to focus on low-level cognitive activities. Employers also do their share of stunting individual skill development. Instead of being equal opportunity employers, most supervisors assign people with disabilities to dead-end, low-paying jobs.

The final result is people with disabilities who fit the negative stereotypes discussed in earlier chapters.

THE QUEST FOR ACCEPTANCE

Within aggregates of persons with disabilities, however, are individuals who have various needs. Some of them have a *dependency need*, which is characterized by dependence on persons in positions of authority for succor. Others have a *status need* as exemplified by seeking recognition from nondisabled persons. The *dominance need* manifests itself in expressions of intellectual superiority. Still others clearly exhibit a combination of these needs. In order to succeed in the larger community, they usually learn to be overtly cooperative, covertly competitive, and publicly inconspicuous. In most instances, success means being accepted as peers by people who do not have disabilities.

Acceptance by significant others builds a positive self-concept, while rejection builds a negative one. Succinctly, *self-concept* refers to the composite of attitudes, beliefs, and values that persons hold pertaining to themselves and the interrelating environmental forces. The self-concept determines an individual's reaction to other people and is shaped by their reaction to him or her. People who feel abused, neglected, or rejected tend to abuse, neglect, or reject other people, including their parents and relatives. Power seems to be a strong antecedent or predictor of the direction of self-concept changes. Individuals high in group or organizational power tend to have positive self-concepts, while those who feel powerless have low self-concepts.

Individuals with disabilities who have a high need for achievement generally set goals of moderate difficulty so that they will succeed. For example, instead of setting a goal of getting a job commensurate with his or her college education, a person who has epilepsy sets his or her sights on getting a job as a clerk. The major emphasis is placed on the highest level of failure. This method of competing with their age-mates for employment is common among persons with disabilities. The fear of failure looms large in their minds. Internal dialogue that reflects the self-conception of a person with a disability includes these questions:

"What type of person am I?" "How do I compare with the other persons?" "What do my friends think of me?" Answers to these questions affect the continuity of his or her mental functioning. Positive or negative responses tell the person: "This is what I am." "This is how I compare with others." "This is what my friends think of me."

Personality theorist Richard Lazarus (1961) noted that adjustment to life situations is always taking place because social, psychologic, and biologic needs are constantly changing. In addition, the environment is constantly changing, and this requires additional adaptive behavior. Change and the subsequent need to adjust to those changes are an integral and natural part of living. Alan Coulter and Henry Marrow (1978) refer to the manner in which people respond to change as *coping*. R. Douglas Whitman (1980) states that coping styles are pathological only if an individual uses excessive psychic energy to cope and distorts reality in the process.

Some of the responses of individuals with disabilities are appropriate; others are not. Furthermore, a response that is appropriate at one time may be totally inappropriate at another time, even under similar circumstances. If every day were the same as the preceding day, very few adjustments would be required. Survival within one's environment would not be a major concern because once a successful adaptation had been made, survival would be insured. However, even though one may wish it, life is not that simple. Each day brings new anxieties and renewed stress situations for all people.

STRESS

Stress and anxiety are feelings all humans experience. *Stress* refers to any assault or demand placed on a person or a system. Stress is often thought of negatively; however, stress *per se* is not harmful. Rather, it is the *reaction to* stress that determines whether it is harmful. Consequently, reactions can produce either good or bad results. Simply stated, stress produces change in emotional state, and each person learns either to tolerate, to reduce, or to eliminate the resultant uncomfortable feelings. If the person fails to respond adequately to stressful situations, his or her behavior may be considered psychologically unsafe. On the other hand, successful adaptation to stress or management of the stressful situation leads to personal growth.

Each person with a disability reacts to stressful situations differently. In fact, what is stressful for one person may not be stressful for another. Lazarus explained what happens when an individual's reactions or adjustment efforts are not successful: "The processes of adjustment are, therefore, important to us not only because under normal circumstances of living they determine our actions but also because when they fail under conditions of unusual demands, our welfare is in danger. When this happens we talk about the existence of a state of stress, an extreme instance of disturbed equilibrium" (p. 303).

All people strive to maintain a balance in their lives, and the struggle for equilibrium occurs at both the conscious and subconscious levels. As an example of the conscious level, many people attempt to keep a proper balance between their social activities and work activities. Simultaneously, their subconscious tries to maintain a balance in emotions. Thus, people may become very elated over an event or find something extremely amusing, but their subconscious will not allow them to remain in an extreme state of euphoria. If they do, the behavior is labeled *abnormal.* Likewise, when they become depressed or unhappy, generally they do not remain in this state for extended periods either. If they do, the behavior is considered psychotic. When people do not return to a state of equilibrium, they experience severe emotional or psychological problems. Lee Sechrest and John Wallace, Jr., (1967) pointed out that most people try to minimize immediate discomfort.

The home is the primary source of security and emotional support or, conversely, stress for most persons with disabilities. A close-knit family is an effective insulation against stress. However, no family can effectively thwart the stress that an individual carries around in his or her subconscious, nor can the individual. Unless one is aware of the origins of a stressful situation, resolution is unlikely.

Stress is psychologically and physically draining on an individual's energies. Some stressful situations are accompanied by considerable physical pain. Louis Kaplan (1965) documented the fact that sociopsychological disorders are not less real or less painful than physical injuries. In fact, psychological stress is more painful to most persons with physical disabilities than their physical impairments. Under conditions of extreme psychological stress, some of them experience adrenal production of desoxycorticosterone, which greatly reduces excitability of the nervous system. The result of desoxycorticosterone production is depression, apathy, and feelings of fatigue and weakness. The gastrointestinal system also responds to stress. For example, a socially or psychologically frightening situation may cause vomiting, nausea, or diarrhea.

During periods of anger, acid production doubles, and heartburn and ulcers are common. The bowel and the stomach are good indicators of how stressful a psychological situation is. Outwardly calm individuals often are burning and churning inside. Other important areas are the cardiovascular and respiratory systems. During conditions of extreme stress, the heart functions in an exaggerated manner; the diaphragm is flattened and shortened, causing cramps in the chest and the inability to take a deep breath. Constant tension in the circulatory system can cause headaches as well as arteriosclerosis. The most serious effect of tension to the cardiovascular system is the formation of blood clots in the heart or brain. It is well known among medical practitioners that excessive stress can lead to asthma, rhinitis, and other allergic symptoms. The mucous membranes of the nose, mouth, throat, and upper respiratory system are extremely sensitive to psychological stress.

Numerous writers, including Charlene DeLoach and Bobby Greer (1981), observed that individuals with disabilities are more vulnerable to anxiety than persons without them. The potential stress is greatly enhanced for individuals with disabilities because the environment has many barriers or restrictions that also create stressful situations. Depending upon the severity of his or her disability, an individual may encounter stress associated with getting an education, participating in social events, securing access to buildings, dating and marriage, and obtaining gainful employment. These overt restrictions, added to numerous covert ones, create frustration and more stress for people with disabilities. James

Sawrey and Charles Telford (1975) summarized these causes of stress in the following manner:

> The person with a disability is more likely to engage in fewer and simpler activities and functions in a more limited area. The restriction is dictated partly by the nature of the disability, but also partly is the result of social attitudes and cultural expectations. When any person has many things done for him, when he does not have to use his own initiative and when his social relations are limited and stereotyped, he has less opportunity and motivation for free and adventuresome idealism and activity. People who could learn to feed themselves are often spoon fed, both literally and figuratively, for many unnecessary years. Socially engendered fearfulness and low levels of self-expectancy promote excessive dependency on others. [P. 70]

Just as persons with disabilities are more vulnerable to stressful situations than persons without disabilities, a person with a disability is more likely to react inappropriately. The reason for this is that social conditioning and the more limited responses available to the individual with a disability compound stressful situations. The unfortunate truth is that many of the appropriate ways of responding to stressful situations are not available to people with disabilities or, at best, are difficult for them to act out. Consider the case of a man who is capable of working (an important factor in establishing positive self-esteem) but is unable to do so because no employer will hire him.

This problem is partially created by societal attitudes that make it not only easy but also acceptable for employers to view a disability as one of the worst things that can happen to an individual. Most workers with disabilities can do much to improve their job skills but very little to alter the negative attitudes of some employers. Too often an employer's solution to the employment problem is to "help" persons with disabilities by providing charity and otherwise protecting them. When a society expects little productivity from people, however, it usually gets little in return. Moreover, those who refuse to be cared for as charity cases experience an inordinate amount of stress.

Methods of Coping

Although persons with disabilities as a group experience stressful situations more often and more intensively than persons without disabilities, the same methods of coping are used by both groups. *Coping mechanisms* are emotions and behaviors that allow an individual to adjust to problems. The survival of all people is dependent on their being able to regulate personal feelings, beliefs, and actions so that their anxiety remains at a manageable level.

There are three categories of coping or defense mechanisms: deception, substitution, and avoidance. Mechanisms of *deception* alter or hide an individual's perception of a threat so that he or she does not sense it. These mechanisms include repression, projection, and displacement. Mechanisms of *substitution* replace stressful goals with those that are safe and relatively tension free. Examples of these mechanisms include compensation and reaction formation. Mechanisms of *avoidance* — those that enable people to remove themselves psychologically from threatening situations — include fantasy and regression.

Sigmund Freud (1938) defined *defense mechanisms* as unconscious, self-deceptive defenses against anxiety. However, Sawrey and Telford stated that it is the motivation behind an act rather than the act itself that is unconscious, for individuals using defense mechanisms may be aware of what they are doing but unaware of the motivation. As noted earlier, individuals with the same disability may not utilize the same defenses because what is stress for one person may not be for another. Also, there is a wide variety of factors that can influence an individual's coping styles, e.g. age at the time of the disability, sex, severity of the disability, and visibility of the disability.

For example, a male who has had polio that leaves him with a limp and one leg smaller than the other will experience less stress dealing with his disability than a female with the same disability and limitations. The reason is that the male can always wear pants in public to hide the leg, whereas a female is likely to encounter situations in which it is more socially acceptable for her to wear a dress, e.g. to church and formal dinners. Also, the appearance of a female's legs probably will be a factor in her overall physical attractiveness, and a limp will draw attention to her leg and thus devalue her appearance.

With respect to age at the time of the disability, a person born with a disability handles stress quite differently than an adult recently disabled. The person born with a disability or acquiring one early in life has not developed a strong nondisability identity that will have to be rethought and reshaped. Conversely, a recently disabled adult has a self-concept much more based on body image and, therefore, a more difficult adjustment.

The rest of this chapter consists of a discussion of defense mechanisms commonly used by persons with (and without) disabilities. The order of their listing should not be interpreted as the order in which they are employed, nor should the reader assume that one defense is more likely to be used than another or than others not mentioned. The major purpose of the discussion is to illuminate several coping styles.

Depression

Depression is a common defense reaction to loss of a body function; however, not all persons experiencing a physical loss immediately become depressed. When depression does occur, individuals generally become despondent over things they can no longer do or those they think they cannot do. Beatrice Wright (1960) refers to *depression* as mourning a loss of a function or a limb no longer available. Often, depression coincides with discovery that limitations are associated with the disability. An individual may become depressed because he or she feels that there is little chance of being independent and that his or her dreams for the future have been shattered, if not destroyed. This form of depressed thinking occurs because the individual continues to cling to the past and has not adapted to the new situation. Individuals who immediately become depressed experience their first serious bout with depression long before they enter the physical rehabilitation stage. Early or late, depression usually is part of the realization that returning to "normal" is going to be impossible or a long and difficult process. It is at this time that the person with disabilities comes face-to-face with reality.

IMPLICATIONS FOR THE REHABILITATION PROCESS. To say that depression is a state of mind that recurs is to state the obvious. However, this statement deserves attention because clients with disabilities have additional stressful situations during rehabilitation about which they seem to be able to do nothing except become depressed. While people with disabilities are in a state of depression, any progress made in the rehabilitation process will at best be limited; however, there are several things that need to be discussed with them during this period: (1) what is psychologically hurting them, (2) how they feel about themselves, (3) what their goals are, what they think they can do, and (4) what lies ahead for them in rehabilitation.

These discussions probably will have to be repeated several times. If an individual is in a state of deep depression, he or she may not hear, or at least not give much attention to, what is being said. Therefore, reinforcement is very important. Even though it may appear that the person is not adequately responding, it is wise to continue communication efforts. Questions oriented to the present and future may gradually shift the individual out of the past. In human relations jargon, this is the process of focusing on the here and now (present) rather than the there and then (past). Leaving the past may not relieve the depression, but it will change it to a different and more manageable form.

Denial

There are two major forms of denial: rationalization and reaction formation. *Rationalization* is the process by which people justify their behavior by replacing the true reasons for it with reasons that are more ego satisfying. The person who rationalizes usually is not trying to distort the truth and is quite unaware of doing so. Rationalization serves to justify what a person thinks, does, and believes. There are several forms of rationalizations; the two that are most relevant to this discussion are "sour grapes" and "sweet lemon."

Devaluing something, for example saying that an unattainable goal is not worthy of interest, is called sour grapes. A person who explains not being hired for a job he or she wanted by saying, "I was glad I didn't get the job after I heard that the company is racist" is demonstrating sour grapes. Sweet lemon rationalization is the opposite, finding something worthwhile in a situation that is undesirable: "Since I have been deaf and learned to read lips, I pay more attention to people. I observe their body language, and so, since being disabled, I understand people better."

Reaction formation is a special type of substitution. This occurs when the original activity is heavily laden with social sanctions and guilt feelings. The person who fears being permanently impaired but jokes about his or her disability and the rehabilitated person who denounces the helpless cripples of the world are exhibiting reaction formation.

IMPLICATIONS FOR THE REHABILITATION PROCESS. After overcoming the shock of discovering that they have a disability, many individuals with permanent disabilities then move to an equally dangerous mind game: denying that they are likely to be physically impaired for the rest of their lives. When people refuse to accept the reality of their disabilities, they often exhibit unproductive behavior such as trying a number of unproven remedies and miracle cures. They become easy marks for unscrupulous con artists who prey on distraught people in order to make money. People in this frame of mind are difficult to assist in the rehabilitation process. They do not want to take on the roles of persons with disabilities restoring themselves to a productive life but instead believe that with one more nontraditional and non–medically proven treatment they will find the cure that will make them "whole" again.

If not carried to an extreme, denial can be beneficial in the rehabilitation process. Sawrey and Telford (1975) observed that, if it is not excessive, denial can help a disabled person to regain his or her psychological equilibrium: "Following the initial period of denial there normally occurs the emergence of a more realistic attitude toward disability. This more realistic and accepting attitude requires an integration of the previous nondisabled self and roles with the individual's changed status. One personality trait that has been shown to be related to this transition is tolerance of ambiguity" (p. 325). Professional and paraprofessional helpers must be alert for denials such as rationalization. Clients may rationalize their lack of initiative by saying that the rehabilitation professionals and paraprofessionals are the experts and know what is best. Through rationalization, they may try to get others to make decisions for them.

Repression

Repression is an unconscious process wherein painful, distasteful, or guilt-producing memories are removed from awareness. An example of repression is the difficulty that might be experienced by a man who as a child was severely beaten by his father for exploring a female playmate's sex organs, when he attempts to explain why he balks at discussing sexual intercourse with his therapist.

IMPLICATIONS FOR THE REHABILITATION PROCESS. Individuals who repress unpleasant thoughts should be encouraged to discuss them. Failure to do so will not only stall or prevent emotional development with regard to their disabilities but also will negatively affect other aspects of their lives in which disabilities have minimal or no impact. As R. Douglas Whitman (1980) pointed out, "Repression can create a snowball effect, as time passes and new things occur which might be associated with anxiety provoking thoughts, these new events and thoughts also must be repressed" (p. 152). The old adage that one cannot solve what one does not know is true. A problem is a puzzle, and repressed thoughts are missing pieces of the rehabilitation puzzle. However, the authors give one final caution: Only well-trained persons should encourage individuals to open up painful, repressed thoughts.

Projection

The process of shifting the responsibility for an act or thought from oneself to another person is called *projection*. This enables an individual to avoid dealing with his or her failures or aggression. For example, a woman who loses her hearing does not admit that she dislikes people who have disabilities but instead cites their hatred and jealousy of her. (It is especially difficult for individuals who were previously able-bodied to accept having a disability.)

IMPLICATIONS FOR THE REHABILITATION PROCESS. Persons with a disability are a product of their environment. Individuals who were not born with a disability but acquired one probably share many of the negative perceptions of people with disabilities that are commonly held by the nondisabled. Now that they, too, are disabled, "one of them," they may project their previous (nondisabled) feelings about disabilities to those around them. Regardless of the fact that their disabilities may not create severe limitations, the knowledge that they no longer are, in their opinion, physically whole causes many persons to ascribe negative attitudes to individuals trying to help them.

Helpers must be aware that people may project an impulse that is threatening onto someone else and attribute it to the external world rather than to themselves. Much of a helper's time and energy may be devoted to getting people with disabilities to own their feelings—getting them to send "I" messages instead of "you," "those people," "them," and "the system" messages. Only by accepting responsibility for their feelings can they gain control of their rehabilitation.

Displacement

Displacement is the process by which an individual releases energy associated with a specific individual or thing onto a secondary target. Displacement is occurring when a woman who is upset with her whining husband who has a disability, instead of confronting him, scolds her children. The reason is quite simple: The children are less threatening than her husband and less able to retaliate. In this situation, it is likely that both the wife and the children will be upset with the husband/father. The process of scapegoating is common in homes where persons with disabilities are protected from ill feelings.

IMPLICATIONS FOR THE REHABILITATION PROCESS. Anger, frustration, fear, and hostility are a few of the emotions felt by persons with disabilities and their loved ones as they attempt to deal with their problems. In many cases people do not know whom to blame for their disabilities; thus, the release of negative emotions usually is directed at the people around them—spouse, parents, siblings, friends, and medical and rehabilitation staff. This scatter-gun approach of dispensing hostile feelings is indiscriminate. In some instances, persons with disabilities will displace their anger on themselves, or, stated another way, the anger becomes internalized, and this leads to depression. In the early stages of adjustment to a disability, the individual with a disability frequently vacillates between depression and displacing anger onto others.

An effective method of working with individuals exhibiting this behavior is to confront them about their actions, making them aware of what the displacement is doing to the people around them and to themselves. A disability does not give an individual license to be insensitive to others or cruel to them. Sometimes people blindly lash out at others because of their own pain, not from malicious intent. However, not even pain absolves them of incivility. Furthermore, assessing blame is seldom helpful. Sometimes, in addition to rehabilitation of the body, there also must be rehabilitation of interpersonal relations.

Sublimation

By channeling energy from prohibited goals or desires to socially acceptable ones, people move one step closer to normalcy. Examples of this process are exercising instead of fighting with a spouse, painting instead of breaking dishes, and lifting weights instead of having sexual intercourse with a friend's girl friend.

IMPLICATIONS FOR THE REHABILITATION PROCESS. Anger and aggression channeled into constructive activities are integral aspects of all rehabilitation programs. A danger, however, is that the displaced activities could replace interaction with people. No amount of exercising, painting, or lifting weights, for example, is an adequate substitute for resolving conflicts between people. There is a tendency to avoid encounters if they have embodied socially unacceptable thoughts. Yet, this is the stuff out of which rehabilitation takes shape. People making is seldom without risks.

Aggression

Aggression can be defined as the first attack or act of hostility, an offensive action. Hostility can be directed inward or outward. Battered and abused children and spouses are but one example of inappropriate, outward-directed aggression.

IMPLICATIONS FOR THE REHABILITATION PROCESS. To make sense of aggression as a coping style, *hostile aggression* and *aggressive behavior* must be distinguished. Hostile aggression serves no useful purpose in the rehabilitation process, and in reality it is a disruptive force that can undo progress that has been made. On the other hand, aggressive behavior can be either productive or unproductive. Aggressively pursuing a rehabilitation program is quite different from hostile aggression.

Aggression is the opposite of passivity, and just as there are times when passive behavior is appropriate, so there are times when being aggressive is the correct behavior. Certainly, there are times when aggressive behavior means asserting oneself. In the case of some people with disabilities, assertive behavior often is not only a desired response but also actively encouraged by rehabilitation personnel.

Dependency

A brief definition of *dependency* is relying on someone or something for help in carrying out activities of daily living. This is the "poor little helpless me" attitude and corresponding behavior. Dependency is a natural state. Whether or not they admit it, all people are dependent on other people to some degree. As the saying goes, "No person is an island," which simply means that no one is capable of meeting 100 percent of his or her needs without help. In fact, even with help, all needs are not met. People need assistance in a variety of areas; therefore, throughout their lives they continually move in and out of stages of dependency.

There is a tendency for most people to think of being dependent in negative terms: Dependent people are sometimes considered lazy, lacking initiative, and possessing very little character. However, what is really being referred to when negative connotations are attributed to dependency is the group of people that Lee Sechrest and John Wallace (1967) refer to as "those who have abandoned attempts to solve their problems and have entrusted the solution of the problems to others" (p. 321). Frequently, persons with disabilities bait this trap by presenting themselves to rehabilitation personnel with a disclaimer of their ability to do anything about their problems, and they catch lots of rehabilitation personnel with this posture.

IMPLICATIONS FOR THE REHABILITATION PROCESS. Rehabilitation personnel and others trying to assist individuals with disabilities must not allow physical disabilities to cloud their vision and distort the helping process. In short, they should not allow persons with disabilities to become overly dependent on them. A balance must be kept between assisting and controlling. One must not lose sight of the ultimate goal in working with the disabled: helping them to help themselves.

Sympathetic emotions are aroused in most people when they see someone whom they believe to be less fortunate than themselves. No matter how noble these feelings are, a person with a disability does not need sympathy. *Sympathy* implies feeling sorry for someone. People with disabilities are capable of producing enough sorrow for themselves; they should be spared additional doses. What they need, and it is in short supply, are empathetic feelings. *Empathy* implies an appreciation of another person's feelings or life situation. Without empathy, rehabilitation becomes an abortion in the helping process: Weak and budding relationships die prematurely.

Self-abasement

Self-abasement is a passive coping mechanism of which the major characteristic is humbling and denigrating oneself. This is a frequently used survival technique, and it is a viable mechanism for several reasons: (1) Persons with disabilities need assistance from others, and one of this society's unspoken norms is that in order to receive help people should humble themselves. (2) As discussed in earlier chapters, many people believe that a disability is the result of sin; therefore, self-abasement is retribution. (3) In some cases individuals with disabilities believe that they are inferior to other people.

IMPLICATIONS FOR THE REHABILITATION PROCESS. It is important that individuals helping people with disabilities do not engage in actions that further devalue them. The old adage, "Beauty is in the eye of the beholder," is certainly appropriate. *Disability* is not a synonym for *ugliness* or *ineptness*. Much of the helper's energies initially may have to be spent accentuating the positive attributes of the person being helped before focusing on behavior that needs change. In the end, rehabilitation will succeed or fail based on the ability of a person with a disability to accept himself or herself as a human being of equal worth and dignity.

Regression

Regression is the mechanism of relieving anxiety or stress by reverting to thoughts, feelings, and behavior that worked well during an earlier period of life. When under mild stress, some adults engage in childlike playing. In extreme stress, they regress to an infantile stage and become unable to wash or feed themselves or control their excretion.

IMPLICATIONS FOR THE REHABILITATION PROCESS. Regression is an attempt to deny reality by distorting it. Helpers may be perceived as parents or lovers or friends who met the person's needs several years ago. While it may be ego gratifying to be considered able to replace an individual's significant others, this does little to cement present relationships. By not accepting helpers for themselves, the person also fails to accept his or her disabilities for what they are. Regression is analogous to taking a detour when going on a mission; it may be interesting and even fun, but it delays the mission.

Compensation

Compensation is the process of enhancing one's self-esteem by excelling in one area to cover up weakness or failure in another. Some people with physical disabilities, for example, become academic achievers in order to compensate for their physical impairments. One of the authors of this book had polio in his right leg at age seven months, which resulted in that leg being shorter and weaker than the left leg. To compensate for difficulty encountered when walking up stairs, he runs up them.

IMPLICATIONS FOR THE REHABILITATION PROCESS. Whether the motivation producing the compensatory act is a feeling of inferiority or a desire to succeed, it is an unconscious decision and must be brought to consciousness. It is helpful for clients to take inventory of themselves in order to know their strengths and weaknesses as well as their coping styles and life goals. Like other defense mechanisms, compensation can be helpful and whole-some when the adjustment is personally and socially beneficial. The first step is, of course, self-knowledge.

Fantasy

The ability to substitute imaginary activities for real ones al-lows some people with physical disabilities to hang on to fragile lifelines, but DeLoach and Greer (1981) took exception to the statement that there is nothing wrong with fantasy. Like the other defenses, there is something very wrong when fantasy is continuous.

IMPLICATIONS FOR THE REHABILITATION PROCESS. All people spend a portion of their lives in fantasy places. The fictitious world of the imagination is certainly a safe haven for persons with disabilities, but this form of flight does nothing to relieve the stresses and barriers in the real world. Fantasy is the "what if" and "I wish" portion of a person's existence. However, one should not abandon the real world for fantasy. Helpers must place this mecha-nism of coping in proper perspective. While no defense mecha-nism can in itself solve problems, fantasy may allow an individual to cope until better solutions are found.

Passing

Passing is the process of denying one's difference and attempting to conceal it. This process is most popularly associated with ethnic minorities who have physical appearances approximating Cauca-sians and who live as Caucasians to avoid discriminatory treatment. Technically, passing is not a defense mechanism since it is a conscious behavior. For the person with a physical disability, passing consists of using cosmetic devices, isolation, and not disclosing the disability. Passing extracts a high price. Sawrey and Telford (1975) wrote: "Concealment indicates shame and involves strain. Despite external vigilance and constant work, the person with a disability often cannot get away from his disability. The price of passing is high and the effort is often futile. When a person must constantly be vigilant in order to deny his disability it becomes the central focus of his life. He may resort to partial social isolation in order to help conceal his defect and thus fend off possible discussion" (pp. 71–72).

IMPLICATIONS FOR THE REHABILITATION PROCESS. Rather than deny their limitations, people with disabilities should accept them, not as red badges of courage, but as reality. Those who pass as nondisabled persons are living a lie that tends to multiply and spread to all areas of their lives. Until they have accepted their disabilities, people with disabilities will not be able to build freely on the resources available within and outside themselves. The freeing dimension of acknowledging that "I have a disability" is the beginning of rehabilitation.

Maladjustment

When defense mechanisms cease to relieve stress, people may turn to behavior that is called *maladjustment* or *maladaption*. A few words of caution are in order at this time: There is a thin line between normal behavior and psychotic and neurotic behavior. Except for extreme psychoses, what is normal and what is not normal are difficult to ascertain. Most normal people have periods of maladjustive behavior; most maladjusted people have periods of rational behavior. According to Harry Milt (1960), borderline personality types exhibit the following behavior:

1. *Belligerence* — walking around continuously with a chip on the shoulder, ready to argue or quarrel at the slightest excuse, or even without an excuse
2. *Excessive moodiness* — spells of blues or feeling down in the dumps, feeling a great deal of time that nothing is worthwhile or really matters
3. *Exaggerated worry* — continuous anxiety about nothing at all or entirely out of proportion to the cause
4. *Suspiciousness and mistrust* — a persistent feeling that the world is full of dishonest, conniving people, that everyone is "trying to take advantage of me"

5. *Selfishness and greediness*—lack of consideration of the needs of others, a "what's in it for me" attitude about almost everything
6. *Helplessness and dependency*—a tendency to let others carry the burden, difficulty in making decisions
7. *Poor emotional control*—exaggerated emotional outbursts out of proportion to their cause and/or at inappropriate times
8. *Daydreaming and fantasy*—spending a good part of the time imagining how things could be rather than dealing with them the way they are
9. *Hypochondria*—worrying a great deal about minor physical ailments, experiencing imaginary symptoms of illness

SUMMARY

People with disabilities who are continuously characterized by all or some of the above conditions are desperate, lonely, and cynical. Indeed, they are alienated from themselves and their significant other persons. The anomic aspects of their alienation are fourfold. They believe that (1) community leaders are indifferent to their needs; (2) their living conditions are getting progressively worse; (3) life is meaningless; and (4) their immediate circle of relationships is not supportive or comfortable. The life theme of alienated people includes a preference for fatalism and an orientation to the past. Feeling helpless in an unpredictable world controlled by people who are not disabled, they resort to a "live for today" philosophy that leaves little room for projecting long-range rehabilitation goals. Fortunately, a growing number of agencies are providing psychological services for people with disabilities and their families. Equally fortunate is the fact that most people with physical disabilities are well-adjusted individuals.

NOTE TO HELPERS

Persons with disabilities are, simultaneously, persons with identities apart from their disabilities. They can best cope with their disabilities when their helpers cope with them. The following observations may help helpers to do this:

1. Helpers cannot solve clients' problems, but they may be able to help them solve their own problems.

2. Every client's problems have more than one possible solution.

3. The easiest, least creative response to disabilities is to pretend they do not exist.

4. Every client behaves according to unwritten ethnic group customs and traditions.

5. The family is the most important group in rehabilitation.

6. Client knowledge of scientific aspects of his or her disability may help or hinder adjustment.

7. Humor can help helpers and people with disabilities over rough spots; people must be able to laugh at themselves and with other people.

8. Previous experience with people with disabilities is a valuable asset if it is used as a general guide. However, if viewed as offering *the* correct view of *every* person with a disability, experience (as well as the information in this book) will be a liability.

9. All helpers make mistakes when working with people with disabilities. They should learn from their mistakes and try not to repeat them.

REFERENCES

Coulter, W. Alan, and Marrow, Henry W. *Adaptive Behavior.* New York: Grune & Stratton, 1978.

DeLoach, Charlene, and Greer, Bobby G. *Adjustment of Severe Physical Disability.* New York: McGraw-Hill, 1981.

Freud, Sigmund. *Basic Writings of Sigmund Freud.* New York: Modern Library, 1938.

Kaplan, Louis. *Foundations of Human Behavior.* New York: Harper & Row, 1965.

Lazarus, Richard S. *Adjustment and Personality.* New York: McGraw-Hill, 1961.

Milt, Harry. *How to Deal with Mental Problems.* New York: National Association for Mental Health, 1960.

Sawrey, James M., and Telford, Charles W. *Psychology of Adjustment.* Boston: Allyn & Bacon, 1975.

Sechrest, Lee, and Wallace, John, Jr. *Psychology and Human Problems.* Columbus, OH: Charles E. Merrill, 1967.

Whitman, R. Douglas. *Adjustment: The Development and Organization of Human Behavior.* New York: Oxford University Press, 1980.

Wright, Beatrice A. *Physical Disability: A Psychological Approach.* New York: Harper & Row, 1960.

Additional Readings

Asratian, Ezras A. *Compensatory Adaptations, Reflex Activity and the Brain.* New York: Pergamon Press, 1965.

Barker, Roger G. *Adjustment to Physical Handicap and Illness.* New York: Social Science Research Council, 1958.

Chevigny, Hector. *The Adjustment of the Blind.* New Haven, CT: Yale University Press, 1950.

Coelbo, George V. *Coping and Adaptation.* New York: Basic Books, 1974.

Cower, Emory L. *Adjustment to Visual Disability in Adolescence.* New York: American Foundation for the Blind, 1961.

McGlade, Francis S. *Adjustive Behavior and Safe Performance.* Springfield, IL: Charles C Thomas, 1970.

Milansky, Aubrey. *Coping with Crisis and Handicap.* New York: Plenum Press, 1981.

Rusalem, Herbert. *Coping with the Unseen Environment.* New York: Teachers College Press, 1972.

Shaffer, Laurance F. *The Psychology of Adjustment.* Boston: Houghton Mifflin, 1936.

Tucker, Irving F. *Adjustment: Models and Mechanism.* New York: Academic Press, 1970.

Young, Kimball. *Personality and Problems of Adjustment.* New York: F. S. Crofts, 1940.

Chapter 7

ORGANIZATIONS FOR CHANGE

The problems of people with disabilities are magnified in the cities. Urban dwellers must continually decide how they can take advantage of the greater abundance of consumer goods and services but overcome the disadvantages that often result from industrialization. The perennial problems of dependent families, neglected and maladjusted children, the aged, the sick and disabled, the unemployed, the functionally illiterate, and minority groups seem to have become accentuated in large urban areas. Most researchers agree that the size and impersonality of the city compound these problems and breed despair among the population.

Lured by the dream of a better life, many rural residents with disadvantaged educational and occupational backgrounds migrate to the cities in search of better education, health, employment, and social conditions. Some have found that the prerequisites for urban adjustment are too high, too demanding, and too unpredictable.

In rehabilitation literature, the behaviors of urban and rural people with disabilities have been described in a variety of ways, ranging from scientific to wholly nonscientific. Some hypotheses have stood the test of empirical investigation; others have not. Theories of "opportunity" and "alienation" seem most relevant to understanding people with physical disabilities and organizations created to help them.

OPPORTUNITY AND ALIENATION

Opportunity refers to an appropriate or favorable time or occasion to function as an integral part of the dominant culture, and *alienation* refers to acts of withdrawal or estrangement from the dominant culture.

Opportunity

Deviant or asocial behavior results from a lack of opportunity for people with disabilities to carry out conforming social behavior. Restricted opportunities to conform are a problem, even if the restrictions are imagined. This theoretical position is built on the belief that a person with a disability (1) must have an opportunity to conform to dominant societal demands, (2) must be capable of such conformity, and (3) must be aware of the opportunity to conform. Inherent in this belief is the assumption that, with few exceptions, people with physical disabilities desire to participate in the dominant community and to be accepted there. It is not the achievement motives of people with and without disabilities that differ but their opportunities to plan, work, and win rewards.

Several years ago, Eva Rosenfeld (1959) observed that deviant styles of life usually are initiated as responses to a series of persistently thwarting experiences, not to a single instance or a few instances of denial of opportunity. She was writing about juvenile delinquents, but her observations are applicable to nondelinquents, too. The family is the primary source of frustrating experiences for most people. Minority-group status, gender differences, inadequate schools, and environmental barriers also give rise to them. This position is in accord with Richard Cloward and Lloyd Ohlin's (1960) classic theory of *differential opportunity.*

It is plausible that the main reason for permitting and facilitating people's access to legitimate opportunity structures is to enhance their feelings of self-worth and identity with the dominant community. (*Opportunity* used in this context refers to the wide range of behaviors and relationships available to nondisabled persons.) Again drawing on a classic study of delinquency, Walter Reckless, Simon Dinitz, and Ellen Murray (1956) demonstrated that a positive self-concept based on dominant cultural norms is the best insulator against deviant behavior. Individuals with disabilities must be permitted to learn majority group social roles, since it is only by performing such roles that they develop feelings of belonging and pride in nondisabled groups. Also, the playing of these roles must take place in situations where they experience affective associations, stability, and productivity.

Males with disabilities, for example, must have opportunities to engage in activities that will permit them to be successful playing male roles. The lack of such opportunities has been well documented in rehabilitation journals. Females with disabilities also need opportunities to carry out conforming behaviors. For instance, most illegitimacy among low-income females can be traced to restrictions on their opportunities to develop and maintain stable, monogamous families. The problem is not that they become unwed mothers; rather, it is the extreme limitations on their opportunities to become wed mothers.

Alienation

Robert Merton (1957), Melvin Seeman (1959), and Dwight Dean (1961) were among the first sociologists to define the phenomenon called *alienation*. It includes feelings of *isolation, normlessness,* and *powerlessness,* which emerge respectively out of feelings of *rejection, instability,* and *failure.* Continued rejection leads to isolation; lack of productive patterned activities leads to normlessness; and a series of failures leads to powerlessness. A socially well adjusted person is the recipient of affect, stability, and productivity. It is important to note that many persons with disabilities engaging in deviant behavior are recipients of affect, stability, and productivity *as handicapped persons.* Their problems begin when they try to behave as nonhandicapped persons.

Individuals with disabilities who are the objects of affect from other people not only are able to perceive themselves as being worthy persons but also are able to perceive themselves as being good persons. On the other hand, a lack of affective attachments to persons whom they like leads to feelings of rejection, and this in turn leads to isolation. The high incidences of social pathologies among persons with disabilities suggest that many of them do not feel that they are wanted. Instead, they feel that few persons, if any, really care about them.

The individual with a disability who is able to perceive his or her life space as somewhat stable is less likely to feel normless. Out of stability come familiarity and patterned activity. Unfortunately, for too many persons with disabilities, stability comes from taking on the roles of invalids, cripples, and handicapped. Without community attachments, some youths and adults with disabilities become nomads, moving from neighborhood to neighborhood, not knowing the faces in their new community and forgetting those in the old ones. The growing number of crimes against persons with disabilities suggests that not only are they denied respect but often they are physically assaulted.

Finally, people with disabilities who experience success in tasks that other people also perform are likely to feel productive. In previous chapters, the many indices of failure that define a *physical disability* as a *social handicap* were discussed. Many aspects of living in today's world combine to distort the personal identities of people with disabilities. Rebelling against the ego disintegration that frequently comes from having a disability, many individuals are demanding a fair chance to be somebody. It is too bad they do not know that they already are somebody.

There are various modes of adaptation to alienation. Some individuals *retreat;* they withdraw and refuse to play able-bodied games of education, work, and social adjustment. Dropping out of school, getting hooked on drugs, and spending most of one's waking hours at home are signs of retreat. In some instances, individuals with disabilities become greatly dissatisfied with their "deviant" behavior and seek to *conform* to the standards set by the dominant community. This is detrimental only if the dominant norms require people with disabilities to be helpless dependents or second-class citizens. On the positive side, conformists attend rehabilitation agencies, engage in job training, and otherwise try to get into the mainstream.

Moderately dissatisfied individuals *innovate* by substituting new means to achieve dominant culture goals. Juvenile delinquents and adult criminals are innovators, for example. In this instance, the system often works for persons with disabilities. The criminal justice system, for example, is less harsh on offenders with disabilities. Severe dissatisfaction with community norms causes a few persons to *rebel.* Most who rebel do so in noncriminal but nevertheless variant manners, e.g. becoming Communists or religious freaks. These individuals have no illusion of being accepted in the larger community, and so they substitute new goals.

There is also the possibility that when dominant community

goals lose their holding power and the other means of adjustment are not attractive, life for persons with disabilities becomes a *ritual* in which they are low achievers but honest citizens. In other words, they are neither troublemakers nor ultraconformists. Instead, they merely exist, playing out their time as a faceless mass of poor people. Skid row is full of able-bodied and disabled ritualists, who usually become retreatists.

Peter Berger (1963) listed four autonomous responses to an oppressive environment: accepting it, transforming it, withdrawing from it, or manipulating it. People with physical disabilities have, at various times, used all four approaches. The disabled people's civil rights movement parallels the black Americans' civil rights movement, which relied heavily on tactics of nonviolent confrontation. Generally, however, people with disabilities have not been as adept as blacks in playing organizational games of infiltration and change. They tend to be easily intimidated by bureaucrats and unaware of their rights and privileges in organizations directly affecting their lives.

PROBLEMS OF CHANGE AGENTS AND THEIR CLIENTS

Throughout the years, social agency personnel involved in change have been mainly mainstream activists—middle-class, respectable persons who work through the "proper channels." Human services personnel acting as links between people with disabilities and those without them must deal with conflicts inherent in serving a population that is believed by many to be drastically different from and at the mercy of people without disabilities, who financially support "programs for the handicapped." The most dedicated human services workers identify with the problems and needs of their clients. However, professional workers who overidentify with clients are vulnerable to the charge of being professionally and emotionally immature. Thus, clients with disabilities are likely to find many human services personnel who privately support them but publicly are less obvious in their commitment.

The dilemma faced by professionals in agencies servicing persons with disabilities is similar to that which professionals faced in antipoverty programs of the early 1960s. For example, Neil Gilbert (1970) observed that most antipoverty personnel during that period tried to play a politically neutral role as middlemen between the distributors and the consumers of social services. In that role, they stressed coordination and cooperation and consequently did little to use government funds to disrupt the activities of local agencies. It was a difficult role then, and it is a difficult one today. The interests of people with disabilities frequently do not coincide with those of public agencies, whose major objectives often include maintaining the status quo.

The practitioners' dilemma is clear: If they do not make demands for change, they are perceived by their clients as having sold out to "the system." If they choose to support their clients' demands, they are labeled *troublemakers* by their agencies. Even when entire agencies take on the advocacy role, the result usually is less than optimal for the clients. Daniel Moynihan (1969) described the typical four-stage sequence for a client-advocacy agency:

> First, a period of organizing, with much publicity and great expectations everywhere. Secondly, the beginning of operations, with the onset of conflict between the agency and local government institutions, with even greater publicity. Thirdly, a period of counterattack from local government, not infrequently accompanied by conflict and difficulties, including accounting troubles, within the agency itself. Fourth, victory for the established institutions or at best, stalemate, accompanied by bitterness and charges of betrayal.... Whereupon it would emerge that the community action agency which had talked so much, been so much in the headlines, promised so much in the way of change in the fundamental of things, was powerless. [Pp. 131–135]

Most advocates of change have been rather naive in thinking that established agencies serving people with disabilities will not resist their own destruction or significant alteration. Some enlightened advocates have called for antiestablishment organizations. By traditional standards, these are radical agencies. In order to understand antiestablishment organizations it is important to know what they do. According to Alan McSurely (1967), on the one hand, establishment organizations teach their workers to (1) maintain objectivity and view people with disabilities as "cases," (2) develop commitment to professional associations rather than clients, (3) set up one-way communication flowing from professionals to clients, (4) develop alliances with elected politicians, and (5) create programs that placate clients. On the other hand, the style of antiestablishment personnel involves (1) treatment of individuals with disabilities rather than of cases, (2) personal commitment to positive changes within organizations, (3) two-way communication between helpers and clients, and (4) building networks with a broad range of community and political persons.

A major problem encountered by most helpers in both establishment and antiestablishment agencies is developing organizations that adequately serve their clients. Without more funding and additional agencies, it is likely that only a small percentage of people with disabilities will ever be served, which means that there is a good chance that the needs of most community rebels will not be met. In terms of advocacy, persons with disabilities whose views are likely to be heard are those who fit into the status quo. Those who gravitate toward leadership positions tend to be upwardly mobile persons who are relatively sophisticated about available opportunities for advancement and are motivated to take advantage of them. There is the danger that antiestablishment organizations, as well as traditional ones, will be dominated by individuals with disabilities who are inclined to use the organizations to fulfill personal rather than group goals.

The more effective helpers learn to tailor their personal visions to fit the actual goals of their clients. When clients choose their own direction, the reform activities tend to be more practical. Individuals who become actively involved in social change risk being legally and physically harassed. Some individuals lose their jobs; others lose social status. When these conditions are considered, it is easy to see why there are few persons working for change. Operating on their own, out in the open, using public confrontation tactics, change agents are very visible, very vulnerable, and very unprotected. A person can get hurt this way. Moreover, there is no guarantee that mourners will flock to the funeral or that friends will take care of the family. Even so, a few change agents believe that fighting the system is not *a* way to help the disabled but *the* way to do it. It is on the bodies of these courageous people that others stand to take advantage of the new opportunities they create.

Of course, social practitioners can elect to work within the system, most of them do. The question raised by many persons with disabilities is, "How effective can one be working for social change within existing human services organizations and political parties?" Obviously, the answer depends on the particular organization and the particular political party. Some organizations are more amenable to change than others, but all organizations resist change. Practitioners may play their organizational roles either sincerely or cynically. Erving Goffman (1959) used the term *sincere* to describe individuals who believe in the impression created by their own performance. On the other hand, cynical performers realize that they are putting on an act and are not taken in by it. Individuals who are brokers of change generally play their roles with cynical detachment. They are like the politicians Gordon Tullock (1965) described: "The successful politician is unlikely to adhere to the highest standards of ethics, but he must make a show of doing so" (p. 38). This is a role quite familiar to many social agency personnel. To achieve their personal goals, some overzealous practitioners give clients incorrect information. Yet, by such means they win the esteem and approval of people with disabilities,

Client self-esteem based on false data is essentially different from that based on true data. Some people with disabilities argue that any kind of esteem is better than no esteem at all, but there are other dimensions and variables. Few organizations allow people with disabilities to be themselves or to express their real selves.

Goffman differentiates between "front stage" and "back stage" behaviors. Western societies, contrasted with non-Western societies, are characterized by the use of one language of behavior for informal (back stage) interaction and another language of behavior for formal (front stage) interaction. When back stage, people can relax, drop their front, and speak their mind. Few persons with disabilities drop their front stage "handicapped" behavior while interacting with professional helpers.

Change-oriented people are likely to find that their personal beliefs are not consonant with prevailing societal beliefs about people with disabilities. This is especially stressful for individuals who are employed in traditional organizations. Some individuals boldly set out to clarify to those around them the exact nature and extent of the differences between them. They literally climb on their soap boxes and try to enlighten the masses. The general result is that their associates label them *strange* and *weird.* There is a predictable sequence of events that normally occurs when individuals deviate noticeably from established societal and agency norms. First, their supervisors and peers direct an increasing amount of communication toward them, trying to change their attitude and behavior. If this fails, one after another of their co-workers abandons the perceived troublemakers as hopeless. Gradually, communication ceases. In the end, the would-be change agents are ignored or excluded from organization activities.

Most persons with disabilities who are effective change agents initially blend into their organizations in a relatively nonthreatening manner, saying little and listening a lot. By presenting this front, they are able to gather information that is helpful in planning for change. The value of protective coloration has long been recognized. Saint Paul recommended this strategy in his first letter to the Corinthians:

> I am a free man, nobody's slave; but I make myself everybody's slave in order to win as many as possible. While working with Jews, I live like a Jew in order to win them; and even though I myself am not subject to the law of Moses, I live as though I were, when working with those who are, in order to win them. In the same way, when with the Gentiles I live like a Gentile, outside the Jewish law, in order to win Gentiles. This does not mean that I don't obey God's law, for I am really under Christ's law. Among the weak in faith I become weak like one of them in order to win them. So I become all things to all men that I may save some of them by any means possible. [1 Corinthians 9:19-23]

Often practitioners learn that even this kind of Machiavellian tactic does not work. Besides, there is the danger that one will become the ingratiating person he or she only pretends to be. Whatever change strategy is used, it is important that individuals choose deliberate deception over self-deception.

ORGANIZATIONAL CHANGES

Given the nature of the problems confronting people with disabilities, it is apparent that institutional changes and modifications are needed to prevent increasing alienation, that additional programs are needed to hold the line and not create proportionately more alienated people. The major programmatic thrust should be toward organization change, particularly where this means removing blocks to learning, broadening opportunities for work and leisure time activities, and otherwise helping people with disabilities.

The aim of any program to improve opportunities for people with disabilities and reduce alienation must reward socially acceptable behaviors in order to enhance the self-concepts of the recipients. An important factor that should determine the type of program to be implemented is whether its primary aim is to reduce external or internal conditions that lead to alienation. Whatever their programs, all human services organizations, as subsystems of the larger society, are affected and constrained by forces in the larger society. Even so, there is much evidence to indicate that social welfare bureaucracies operate with a considerable degree of autonomy. Government human services agencies neither depend on nor are controlled by their clients. Some agencies gain so much power that they are not really controlled by either taxpayers or elected officials.

The fact that most human services agencies are not completely controlled by clients, the general taxpaying public, or elected officials does not preclude the possibility that some agency administrators are surrogates for community decision makers. Often the decision about who gets a service or who gets a job is made in consultation with individuals whom Floyd Hunter (1953) called the "power elite." In addition to the power elite, many local agencies are controlled by rules and regulations decided at the state or federal level. An agency's freedom of action may be considerably restricted by such rules. Furthermore, the rules may be so contradictory, so numerous, so complicated, and so changeable that only a few knowledgeable personnel (often clerks) know the latitude of action available to the agency. Little wonder, then, that both clients and their helpers are frustrated from time to time.

Interagency differences are quite noticeable, and these inconsistencies are directly traceable to differences in organization direction.

In short, there are differences in the kinds of goals defined by each agency and in the administrative methods used to achieve them. In an agency whose director is strongly committed to the concept of *human service,* the organization tends to be client oriented and internally permissive. In another agency, which is not visibly different in terms of social and political environment, the director is rule oriented and authoritarian, and the workers are considerably more limited in the services they provide clients.

The examples cited illustrate not only the degree of autonomy an agency may have but also the skewing of power that may exist within it. In many instances, contrary to popular opinion, the attitudes of social practitioners are not a significant variable in service delivery. The fact that human services agencies have power does not mean that it is placed in the hands of their personnel. The average practitioner has little to offer but dedication and limited expertise, and few agency administrators are awed by such resources.

Successfully helping persons with disabilities requires considerable skill in manipulating rules and mobilizing collegial support. Individuals concerned with organizational change should ask themselves the following questions:

1. What do I want?
2. Which of my goals for change are most important?
3. What power do I have to bring about change?
4. What possible allies and other sources of power might I be able to tap?
5. What might happen to limit the power I have or may be able to tap?
6. What is the organization most likely and least likely to change?
7. How can I move from plans to action?

It is important for practitioners to use tactics appropriate to their roles. Also, the issues and forces (facilitating and restraining) must be adequately researched. Again, would-be change agents should not be surprised when the system fights back. Still, throughout the years there have been some remarkable changes in private and public agencies serving people with disabilities.

There is a long list of role models for Americans who aspire to create and improve organizations dedicated to helping people with disabilities. Included in the list are Dorothea Dix, who led the drive to improve mental hospitals in the United States; the Reverend John Stanford, who established the New York Institution for the Deaf and Dumb in 1818; Samuel Howe, who in 1832 founded what became the Perkins Institution for the Blind; and Edgar Helm, a Methodist minister who founded the Goodwill Industries of America in 1902.

Most private organizations that help people with disabilities began with a few persons speaking out and attracting supporters who held similar views. The joining together of individuals with similar interests has led to the formation of associations that focus on specific disabilities, e.g. the Epilepsy Foundation of America, the Arthritis Foundation, the United Cerebral Palsy Association, the National Multiple Sclerosis Society, the Juvenile Diabetes Foundation, the National Society for the Prevention of Blindness, the National Association of the Deaf, and the Cystic Fibrosis Foundation. (A more complete list is provided in Appendix B.) As these agencies have matured, they have changed and tried to be more responsive to their clients.

Nationally, there is a new spirit of change among human services agencies. Administratively the changes are being championed by a new breed of directors, those who dare to innovate, risk public ridicule, and deviate from tradition in order to solve rehabilitation problems. The rigid conformists and the technocratic midgets are on the way out. Therefore, the earlier concept of rigid structures and inept practitioners is slowly giving ground to a picture of human services personnel with a desire and will to be more effective helpers. This change is vividly seen in leisure-oriented programs.

Leisure-Oriented Programs

Even when people with disabilities are able to get high-paying jobs, their struggle to fit into the mainstream usually does not end. During the last decade, technology has reduced the labor time of many workers with disabilities from fifty hours per week to less than forty. This leisure time quite often is used for recreation.

This is best illustrated by the many motor homes seen on the highways, especially during the summer months. Almost every large city is in the process of building or has built nature trails for hikers. Lakes, camping grounds, and amusement parks continue to be developed and expanded in order to capture the increasing numbers of persons who avail themselves of their services.

Fortunately, people with disabilities and those concerned with their welfare have taken steps to ensure that they have opportunities to participate not only in work but also in play. Just as builders of homes and commercial structures have been made aware of the need for barrier-free buildings, builders of recreation facilities are responding to the request for wider spaces for handicapped parking, curb cuts, rails in bathrooms, wider doors and aisles that will accommodate wheelchairs, and lower booths, water fountains, and tables that will allow a person in a wheelchair to gain access. Approximately two dozen national agencies and organizations have been developed specifically to assist in providing recreation and/or recreation information and assistance for persons with disabilities. Many more local and state organizations exist to provide similar services. Even so, most recreation facilities are not accessible to persons with disabilities.

In preparing for a vacation or a recreational outing, generally the first step is to plan for places to visit. Not knowing whether facilities are accessible serves as a source of frustration to people with disabilities. Every state has at least one travel information center that provides information about accessibility to local recreation facilities. More specific to those with physical disabilities is the information provided by the Travel Information Center of the Moss Rehabilitation Hospital in Philadelphia, Pennsylvania. People with physical disabilities who inquire of this Center receive information such as hotels and motels that have wheelchair ramps, and airlines and cruise ships that make every reasonable effort to accommodate those with physical disabilities. The Center also lists countries and cities that accommodate visitors with disabilities and historical sites, tourist attractions, public facilities, national monuments, and other points of interest to visitors that are accessible to people with physical disabilities.

By purchasing a membership in certain organizations, individuals with disabilities receive travel information designed to eliminate or minimize the hazards of travel. AWill/AWay RVer's Association and Mobility International U.S.A. are examples of such organizations. AWill/AWay RVer's provides travel information to disabled persons who travel in recreational vehicles. Mobility International U.S.A. is an affiliate of Mobility International, a British organization founded for the purpose of providing people having disabilities with information about travel and leisure opportunities as well as educational opportunities. Other organizations, such as Ability Tours and Evergreen Travel Service, provide information about accessibility and accommodations and also plan and provide tours for travelers with disabilities. If transportation is by commercial airplane, Access to the Skies provides information regarding airlines that accommodate young and old travelers. This organization also provides assistance to airlines in making their aircraft accessible to persons with physical disabilities.

Some national organizations, such as the Boy Scouts and Girl Scouts of America and the National Red Cross, have expanded their services in order to enable persons with disabilities to participate. In several instances, individuals with disabilities have founded their own organizations to provide for recreational activities, e.g. the American Blind Bowling Association, the American Athletic Association for the Deaf, the National Wheelchair Athletic Association, and the National Wheelchair Basketball Association. (A list of additional resources for recreation is found in Appendix C.)

It is a sign of progress that people with disabilities are focusing on accessibility of recreation. This does not mean that job discrimination, segregation in housing, and inadequate education are no longer problems, however. Rather, it means that people with disabilities have expanded their social action agenda to take steps necessary to bring them closer to other citizens in all opportunities.

UTILIZATION OF RESOURCES

A major problem in getting services to people with disabilities is the agencies' geographical location and utilization patterns.

Almost every disability has an association or foundation charged with the responsibility of sponsoring research about it and fostering services for it. In addition, there are a variety of non–disability-oriented organizations that offer related or complementary services. In some cases it is this large maze of organizations through which people with disabilities or their advocates have to go in order to be helped. The fact that there are several organizations with similar names and similar services adds to the consumers' confusion.

Another major problem many people have is not knowing what resources are available. It may seem strange that with such a large number of organizations most persons with disabilities are not familiar with the ones pertaining to them. It must be remembered that, historically, they have been *told* where to go rather than being encouraged to make this decision for themselves. Fortunately, persons with disabilities as a generalizable group no longer are subscribing to the idea that "If I need a service someone will tell me I need it and where to get it." They are becoming much more astute at seeking and receiving information. A growing number of them are aware that the federal government and most states have information services listed in telephone directories. Also, they are becoming aware that an excellent place to start in the search for appropriate services is a vocational rehabilitation office.

Any community program undertaken to improve opportunities for people with disabilities and reduce their alienation must reward socially acceptable behaviors. Also, based on individual needs, there must be a wide variety of programs. For example, personality disturbances can best be ameliorated in agencies that provide individual treatment; intergroup conflict is within the purview of human rights organizations; educational deficiencies are problems for schools. Each agency is part of a gestalt in which the whole is greater than the individual parts. It is important for the disabled to see and understand the total community resources available to help them. Finally, the more effective programs are those in which the people served are actors and not merely objects acted upon.

Programs designed primarily for the institutionalization and containment of persons with disabilities are inferior to those which permit individual growth and development. Any agency or program that is capable of helping people to succeed or fail on their abilities is vastly superior to those in which they must passively await the capricious or paternalistic and maternalistic decisions of their helpers.

RECOMMENDATIONS

The following minimum community activities are basic to the curtailment of alienation:

1. Existing disability-oriented agencies should be expanded, and new opportunities for people with disabilities should be created. This may require adjusting agency programs to meet new needs.

2. Remedial programs should be provided to prepare unqualified clients to utilize existing opportunities and be prepared for future opportunities.

3. Counseling programs should be expanded to raise the educational and occupational aspirations of persons with disabilities to a sufficiently high level and keep them there, in order not to channel them into cultures of poverty.

4. Provisions for rewarding approved behaviors should be built into agency services. Such rewards could include verbal praise, more difficult tasks, financial assistance, and timely terminations.

5. Special programs of leisure-time activities, including those encouraging client self-direction, should be expanded.

6. Periodic surveys should be made in order to evaluate the effectiveness of existing services and point out gaps in total services. It is imperative that stratified samplings of the disabled population be used in such surveys.

SUMMARY

The authors cannot emphasize enough the fact that the school, rehabilitation, and other community resources must be relevant, available, and known. The more effective programs are those with a well-trained, dedicated staff. Also, by working cooperatively with other agencies, they are able to avoid needless duplication of personnel and financial resources. Because these programs are "helping" and "enabling" programs, their major focus is getting people with disabilities into the dominant culture as first-class citizens.

NOTE TO HELPERS

Group membership is a primary source of security (or insecurity) for the individual. Because groups serve as the foremost determiners of self-esteem, feelings of worth depend upon the social status of the groups to which a person belongs. It should not be surprising, therefore, that persons with disabilities who believe they are members of low-status or underprivileged groups tend toward feelings of self-hatred and worthlessness. Merle Ohlsen (1970) lists several characteristics of an effective group. The most important characteristic is that the members must cooperate to achieve common goals. This means that the group—

1. knows why it exists.
2. has created an atmosphere in which its work can be done.
3. has developed guidelines for making decisions.
4. has established conditions under which each member can make his or her unique contributions.
5. has achieved communication among its members.
6. has helped its members learn to give and receive help.
7. has learned to cope with conflict.
8. has learned to analyze its processes and improve its functioning.
9. provides a safe place in which its members express their ideas and receive honest reactions from others.

The following specific behaviors aid a group in completing its tasks:

1. *Initiating*—suggesting new ideas or a different way of looking at the group's problems or goals, proposing new activities
2. *Information seeking*—asking for relevant facts or information
3. *Information giving*—providing pertinent facts or authoritative information
4. *Opinion giving*—stating a belief or opinion about something the group is discussing

5. *Elaborating*—building on a previous comment, enlarging on it, giving examples

6. *Coordinating*—showing or clarifying the relationship among various ideas, trying to pull ideas and suggestions together

7. *Orienting*—defining the progress of the discussion in terms of the group's goals, raising questions about the direction the discussion is taking

8. *Testing*—checking with the group to see if it is ready to make a decision or take some action

Disruptive or dysfunctional forms of behavior that impede group movement toward its goals include the following:

1. *Blocking*—interfering with the progress of the group by going off at a tangent, citing personal experiences unrelated to the group's problem, arguing too much on a point the other members have resolved, rejecting ideas without consideration, preventing a vote

2. *Aggression*—criticizing or blaming others, showing hostility toward the group or some individual without relation to what has happened in the group, attacking the motives of others, deflating the ego or status of others

3. *Seeking recognition*—attempting to call attention to oneself by excessive talking, extreme ideas, boasting, and/or boisterousness

4. *Special pleading*—introducing or supporting ideas related to one's own pet concerns or philosophy beyond reason, attempting to speak for "the grass roots," "the masses of people"

5. *Withdrawing*—acting indifferent or passive, resorting to excessive formality, doodling, whispering to others

6. *Dominating*—trying to assert authority in manipulating the group or certain members of it by "pulling rank," giving directions authoritatively, interrupting others

Professionals in organizations should be familiar with the points listed above so that they can facilitate effective organizations. At the very least, professionals should learn to be helpful rather than disruptive group members. Of course, their clients may benefit from this information, too.

REFERENCES

Berger, Peter. *Invitation to Sociology: A Humanistic Perspective.* New York: Doubleday, 1963.

Cloward, Richard A., and Ohlin, Lloyd E. *Delinquency and Opportunity.* New York: Free Press, 1960.

Dean, Dwight G. Meaning and measurement of alienation. *Am Soc Rev, 26:* 753–758, 1961.

Gilbert, Neil. *Clients or Constituents.* San Francisco: Jossey-Bass, 1970.

Goffman, Erving. *The Presentation of Self in Everyday Life.* Garden City, NY: Doubleday, 1959.

Hunter, Floyd. *Community Power Structure: A Study of Decision Makers.* Chapel Hill: University of North Carolina Press, 1953.

McSurely, Alan. *Hangups.* Louisville, KY: Southern Conference Educational Fund, 1967.

Merton, Robert K. *Social Theory and Social Structure.* New York: Free Press, 1957.

Moynihan, Daniel. *Maximum Feasible Misunderstanding.* New York: Free Press, 1969.

Ohlsen, Merle M. *Group Counseling.* New York: Holt, Rinehart & Winston, 1970.

Reckless, Walter C., Dinitz, Simon, and Murray, Ellen. Self concept as an insulator against delinquency. *Am Soc Rev, 21:* 744–746, 1956.

Rosenfeld, Eva. A research-based proposal for a community program of delinquency prevention. *Annals, 21:* 136–145, 1959.

Seeman, Melvin. On the meaning of alienation. *Am Soc Rev, 24:* 783–791, 1959.

Tullock, Gordon. *The Politics of Bureaucracy.* Washington, DC: Public Affairs Press, 1965.

Wright, George N. *Total Rehabilitation.* Boston: Little, Brown, 1980.

Additional Readings

Aldrich, Howard. *Organizations and Environment.* Englewood Cliffs, NJ: Prentice-Hall, 1979.

Dyer, William G. *Insight to Impact: Strategies for Interpersonal and Organizational Change.* Provo, UT: Brigham Young University Press, 1976.

Elder, Jerry O., and Magrab, Phyllis R. (Eds.). *Coordinating Services to Handicapped Children: A Handbook for Interagency Collaboration.* Baltimore: Paul H. Brookes, 1980.

Emener, William G., Luck, Richard S., and Smits, Stanley J. (Eds.). *Rehabilitation, Administration & Supervision.* Baltimore: University Park Press, 1981.

Fairweather, George F. *Creating Change in Mental Health Organizations.* New York: Pergamon Press, 1974.

Grossman, Lee. *The Change Agent.* New York: AMACOM, 1974.

Hultman, Ken. *The Path of Least Resistance: Preparing Employees for Change.* Austin, TX: Learning Concepts, 1979.

Hutchinson, Peggy, and Lord, John. *Recreation Integration: Issues and Alternatives in Leisure Services and Community Involvement.* Ontario, Canada: Leisurability, 1979.

Magrab, Phyllis R., and Elder, Jerry O. *Planning for Services to Handicapped Persons: Community, Education, Health.* Baltimore: Paul H. Brookes, 1979.

Meyer, Marshall W. *Change in Public Bureaucracies.* New York: Cambridge University Press, 1979.

Moran, Robert T., and Harris, Philip R. *Managing Cultural Synergy.* Houston, TX: Gulf, 1982.

Pan, Elizabeth L., Backer, Thomas E., and Vash, Carolyn L. (Eds.). *Annual Review of Rehabilitation: Volume 1, 1980.* New York: Springer, 1980.

Pan, Elizabeth L., Backer, Thomas E., and Vash, Carolyn L. (Eds.). *Annual Review of Rehabilitation: Volume 2, 1981.* New York: Springer, 1981.

Sperry, Len, Mickelson, Douglas J., and Hunsaker, Phillip L. *You Can Make It Happen: A Guide to Self-Actualization and Organizational Change.* Reading, MA: Addison-Wesley, 1977.

Wehman, Paul, and Schleien, Stuart J. *Leisure Programs for Handicapped Persons: Adaptations, Techniques, and Curriculum.* Baltimore: University Park Press, 1981.

Chapter 8

TIPS FOR PARENTS

Each person with a disability must live with his or her disability and adjust to it. Perhaps the most difficult aspect of this process is learning to accept the responses of nondisabled people to the disability. This is especially difficult because there is no foolproof way to predict whether onlookers will display acceptance or rejection. When decoded, a large number of public responses convey rejection, pity, and overprotectiveness. Although caring persons wish that none of these things would happen, realistic persons know that they can and often do happen.

Bette Ross (1981), Robert Perske (1981), and Helen Featherstone (1980) pointed out that the emotions surrounding a physical disability go up and down as if on a roller coaster, moving through remorse, relief, and resolution. In reality a disability is a family condition; it is never a problem of just the person with the disability. Of all the family members, parents are the most affected. In this chapter the authors will use the terms *child* and *children* to mean a person or persons of any age from birth to death, because a child—whatever his or her age—is always a child to his or her parents.

MEMBERS OF THE FAMILY DRAMA

All members of the family are important. However, depending on the situation, some are treated as if they were more important at a given moment than others. Rehabilitation is easier when persons with disabilities and their relatives accept the disabilities without guilt or hostility. Frequently, this requires relatives to leave the physical care to others while they provide emotional care. William Kvaraceus and E. Nelson Hayes (1969) observed that when parents learn of their child's permanent disability they usually pass through three stages. It does not matter if the disability occurs at birth or during late adulthood; most parents do some fairly predictable things.

Stage 1 is the period of trying to find proof that the child is not abnormal or permanently disabled. This consists of taking the child to see several physicians in order to get "the good news" that the disability is temporary and does not impair the individual's functioning. This stage also includes voracious reading about the disability and seeking out other persons who have experienced it. During this stage, there is a frantic search to find someone or something to make the disability go away. While searching for a positive diagnosis, finances are drained in middle-income families and depleted in low-income families.

Stage 2 is the period in which parents are determined to prove that the experts are wrong. This could be called the "pray for miracles" stage. Usually, one parent becomes obsessed with taking care of the child. Gradually, the interaction between spouses changes as the child becomes a wedge. It is not uncommon for one spouse to lose interest in sexual intercourse, refuse to associate with other people, neglect her or his duties within and outside the home, and spend an inordinate amount of time with the child trying to help him or her to be like a "normal" person. It is typical for the consumed parent to convince herself or himself that the child is a misunderstood genius. If there are other children in the family, they begin to feel neglected, and the other relatives begin to feel estranged from the situation. This, then, is the most crucial period in family interpersonal relationships.

Stage 3, if it occurs, is characterized by both parents' accepting the child's disability as being permanent but not a disaster. Often, parental separation or divorce precedes this stage. Only by accepting the disability are parents able fully to accept the child and, relatedly, themselves. It need not be, but it often is, a personally painful and financially costly journey from Stage 1 to Stage 3. Nor is it necessary to go through all three stages. Throughout the entire drama, it becomes clear that family members and the child are persons first and social role players second. Parents in particular tend to forget or not learn this basic fact. Leo Buscaglia (1975) wrote:

"Only in rare instances does becoming a parent drastically change the *person* one is. Most generally, a thoughtful person will make a thoughtful parent. A loving person will be a loving parent. On the other hand, a confused or neurotic person will also make a confused and neurotic parent" (p. 84). There are good and bad actors playing parent roles.

The Mother Role

A woman's concept of the mother role is shaped by the culture and social class in which she lives. Initially, she is likely to respond to maternal cues in the same way her mother or mother surrogate responded to similar cues. The mother role is learned; it is not in the genes. Motherly love can be the strongest emotional tie between two human beings, or it can be the weakest. Most societies ascribe to mothers the nurturing role. Thus, it is expected that mothers will have the responsibility for taking care of their children's emotional needs. Fathers are not unable to do this, but they seldom are conditioned or expected to do it.

In most societies it is expected that two of the primary female roles in marriage are wife and mother; the corresponding male roles are husband and father. The father and mother roles are concerned mainly with providing love and discipline to their children. To do this effectively, some mothers delegate discipline to the father, and some fathers delegate love sharing to the mother. In a balanced marriage, however, mothers and fathers share these responsibilities. There is no valid reason to attribute nurturing behavior to women in their wife and mother roles and discipline behavior to men in their husband and father roles. What is more important in terms of effective parenthood is that there is teamwork in caring for children, especially children with disabilities.

The Father Role

There has been considerably less attention given to father roles. This is the case even though there is a difference between fatherhood and being a father. Like the mother role, the father role is learned. The image of the virile male is believed by many people to be incompatible with tender feelings. To deny fathers their social or individual right to express tenderness and gentleness is to deny them emotions they naturally feel for their children. Some fathers voluntarily deny these feelings, however. In an attempt to wall out "feminine" and tender feelings, some fathers go to great lengths not to show their love. C. S. Lewis (1972) cautioned these persons: "If you want to make sure of keeping your heart intact, you must give it to no one. Avoid all entanglements, lock it up safe in the coffin of selfishness. But in that coffin—safe, dark, motionless, airless—it will change. It will not be broken; it will become unbreakable, and irredeemable" (p. 112).

Because the bonding between most mothers and their children is very strong, the father's role is likely to seem secondary, and he may feel left out. If the child with a disability is male, a father is likely to have conflicting feelings—anger and pity. Females with disabilities are less difficult to accept as dependents. After all, there is little shame in a father's taking care of a daughter, whatever her age. However, sons are expected to take care of not only themselves but also their own families when they grow up.

The Other Family Members' Role

In most cases, the concerns parents have for a child with a disability are family concerns and must be treated as such. It is counterproductive to define the child with a disability as a responsibility only of his or her parents. All members of the family, including extended family members, should be involved in the rehabilitation process. To do this, they must have an accurate understanding of the child's disability and be in touch with their own feelings about the disability and the child. The family members' role in the helping process first begins in handling their own negative feelings of shame, anger, self-pity, hurt, and frustration. Second, they need to learn helpful ways to relate to the child. Throughout this process, care must be taken not to neglect the other family members.

In the end, it is not so much what medical, rehabilitation, and educational personnel do that brings about a satisfactory adjustment to a disability but, instead, what the family does. This is not to say that the family members alone can bring about an effective adjustment. They certainly need the help of friends, professionals, and self-help groups. Nor are family members ever neutral in the rehabilitation process. On the contrary, they are positive or negative catalysts for adjustment.

NORMAL FEELINGS AND BEHAVIORS

Tucked securely somewhere in the minds of most people is the belief that they should not display behavior that indicates feelings of weakness or culpability. Yet, it is the denial of these feelings that renders would-be helpers ineffective when dealing with the disabled. Parents are particularly sensitive to what they believe is the need of their disabled child not to be upset by the negative feelings of others. Alfred Katz (1961), Benjamin Spock and Marion Lerrigo (1965), and Helen Featherstone (1980) provide informative, sensitive views of being parents of a child with a disability. Feelings are neither logical nor predictable: They just are. Some parents make the mistake of singling out other parents whom they admire and then trying to emulate them. Each parent of a child with a disability usually learns how to deal helpfully with his or her feelings not by example but by trial and error experiences. Behaviors that fit one parent may not fit another. Like the helpers described in other chapters of this book, parents must be congruent in their feelings and behaviors, which should be positive toward their children.

Each member of the family, including the person with the disability will feel different about the disability at different times. Whatever their feelings, it is important to discuss them openly and honestly. Admittedly this is easier said than done. There is a danger in open dialogues of this kind. They should not be encouraged if family members will be reprimanded for expressing negative feelings. An open, honest dialogue is just that: It is the way people feel at the time of the discussion. Some parents scold siblings for expressing jealousy or hatred of a brother or sister with a disability. Rather than scolding, it is more helpful to try to find out why they feel the way they do about their sibling. Little is accomplished when parents try to squash expression of these feelings. Besides, with or without approval, they will surface.

It is difficult for most persons to state their negative feelings about a loved one, and it is exceptionally difficult to share negative feelings about a "crippled" family member. Few families openly and honestly deal with any interpersonal problem. Generally, there is a conspiracy of silence when the members are together, and secret character assassination when they are apart. The more productive sharing sessions also include positive feelings. If a family convenes to talk about problems but seldom about feelings of happiness, pride, and positive growth, they will split into unmendable pieces.

Self-pity

Anything that diminishes the social worth of children also damages the egos of their parents, siblings, and other relatives. Pity expressed for the person with a disability often is displacement of deeply felt self-pity. For example, in their solitude, parents may ask: "Why did this terrible thing happen to us? What have we done to be punished this way? What will the neighbors think?" Parental self-pity is heightened by the realization that some of the dreams they had for the child with the disability will not be realized. The young child will not become a candidate for the prettiest baby contest, the teenage child is not likely to become a superstar in sports, and the adult may not be able to have children. (Interestingly, few able-bodied children can make most of their parents' dreams come true either). Exaggerated self-pity can cause parents to view the child as their personal "cross to bear." They become God's self-appointed martyrs.

It is normal to engage in self-pity and to grieve. Most parents wish the best for their children. In many ways, children who have spina bifida, cerebral palsy, loss of hearing or vision, or some other impairment have died a bit. Those parts or functions are lost, and to pretend that they are not will delay or prevent successful rehabilitation. Yet, it is important to remember that children with disabilities are still alive. Sometimes parents talk about them as if they were dead, e.g. "Johnny was so full of life" or "Sue was a joy to be around."

Magic Cures

The desire to cure the child with a disability leads some parents down several false trails, and they run faster when they see children the same approximate age as their child doing things they would like their child to do. There are nagging "what if" thoughts that may even drive parents to seek miracle or magical cures from known charlatans. Dreams of success are not easily abandoned and are seldom forgotten. The quest for cure is accelerated when a child begins to lose control of muscles or limbs or body functions that he or she once had. Also, congenital disabilities often are easier for parents to accept than those resulting from accidents.

It is normal to be shocked and to disbelieve the diagnosis of permanent disability. There are no good ways to prepare oneself or others to accept a disability. However, some ways are less traumatic than others. Understanding the medical aspects of a disability does not lessen the anguish, but it allows one to act from intelligence instead of ignorance. When "what if" is asked, the answer is always the same: No amount of conjecture will alter the fact of the disability. By dwelling on idle speculation, parents and others often overlook an important fact: Most people with permanent disabilities cannot be cured, but they can be kept well enough to function in the larger society. A permanent disability does not *ipso facto* mean a permanent handicap. Indeed, most people with disabilities can be, and usually are, happy and well adjusted. Being permanently disabled is not automatically being relegated to sadness.

Guilt and Shame

Sometimes parents feel guilty when they wish the child with a disability had not been born or wish that he or she were dead. These are not always evil wishes, but they are always conjured up out of feelings of helplessness. Feelings of guilt are not the same as feelings of shame. Guilt is self-centered, and shame is other-centered. Parents who feel guilty are likely to ask what they have done to cause the disability. Parents who feel ashamed worry about what other people—friends, neighbors and other relatives—will think about the disabled child. Excessive shame can lead people to *think* that they are sinful and unworthy of love, while excessive guilt causes them to *know* that they are sinful and unworthy of love.

It is normal to have feelings of guilt and shame. However, it is not normal to have excessive feelings of this nature. Parents of a child with a disability must accept themselves and their child if their home is to be a good environment for all its members. If parents can publicly present their child to others without feelings of excessive guilt or shame, then the child can more easily take pleasure in public activities.

Overprotection

Often guilt gives way to overprotection. "This is my child and nobody is going to abuse him. He may be handicapped but he's my baby," a mother said. Her baby was thirty years old, and she treated him like a ten-year-old. Under most conditions, it is difficult for parents not to smother a child. It is even more difficult when their child has a disability. Smothering weakens parents and their children. It is an act of love to give children room to grow and learn.

It is normal for parents to want to protect their children from physical and emotional pain. How much hurt can parents spare their children? Obviously, parents cannot wish away or stop their children's pain, but they can minimize it. In reality, parents cannot spare children the hurt others will inflict on them, so some parents try to prepare their children for it. One way of doing this is to fully develop each child's abilities. Thus, instead of focusing on what a child cannot do, the more helpful parents focus on what he or she *can* do. The goal of parenting is to prepare children for lives away from their parents. This requires a realistic assessment of each child's skills, abilities, and potential. The following prayer is appropriate for both parents and children: "God grant me the serenity to accept things I cannot change, the courage to change things I can, and the wisdom to know the difference." Unrealistic ambitions lead to needless frustration, while falsely deflated aspirations result in needless mediocrity.

Resentment

Caring for any child is a chore, and caring for a child with a physical disability can be a tedious chore. Overprotection gives way to resentment. Feeling trapped in a series of activities that seem to have no end, parents of a child with a permanent disability often become entombed in their own altruism. This feeling is heightened when friends and funds begin to wane. Sibling problems are likely to become acute when most of the family's time and financial resources are spent taking care of one of its members. Well-intentioned relatives only add to the resentment when they, too, treat the child with a disability as a special person. They forget that *all* children (and adults) should be treated as special persons.

It is normal for parents who spend an inordinate amount of time with their children to feel resentful. It is normal to complain and even cry when they feel overworked and locked into an activity. This feeling is often related to overprotection. The child with a disability should be fit into the family schedule instead of vice versa. Much of the resentment parents feel could be avoided if the child were allowed to be a regular member of the family. Care must be taken not to cause the child with a disability to be physically in but socially out of the family. Prima donnas seldom are "in" with the other actors in a play, and children with disabilities treated like prima donnas seldom are appreciated by other family members.

It is parental love that allows a child to cope with his or her disability as a member of the family. Some parents do not realize that their children need time away from them, too. In order to stay in the family, persons with disabilities must respect themselves and other people and their spaces. Any change in one family member affects the other members, and it is within the family that the child with a disability learns whether or not it is okay to be himself or herself. Much of the time that family members spend with the child is not helpful because it is spent treating him or her like an invalid and not like a person of equal value. The key is to encourage people with disabilities to be independent in most activities and able to ask for help in those requiring assistance.

SELF-DIRECTED CHILDREN

Parents who do not produce self-directed children fail everyone — their children and the society they will serve. The older children become, the more difficult it is for them to learn to be self-directing. The question is, "How can parents produce self-directed children with disabilities?"

First, parents must believe that self-direction is important. Each parent must not simply give lip service to the concept but must be willing to put it to practice in the home. Self-direction should be a living concept; it must be given as much practice as subject matter recitals in school. All children learn by doing, and they learn best by assisting in planning and carrying out their own activities.

Second, parents must trust their children to learn. As noted, too many parents try to protect their children from failure and, consequently, do not give them difficult chores. Responsibility and self-direction are learned. If children with disabilities are going to learn self-direction, then it must be through being given opportunities to succeed and fail in family-related activities. Along this line of thought, if a child believes in his or her own inadequacy or lack of power when confronted with new situations, failure is certain. As a child falls further and further behind his or her peers in skill development, there is a diminishing of his or her self-concept. Parents cannot do a task for a child and develop his or her task mastery. A sense of success comes only from an individual's own task mastery.

Third, parents of a child with a disability need to maintain an experimental attitude. When their child is given the opportunity to try new (or old) behaviors, parents should not be alarmed or disappointed when he or she makes mistakes. Letting children make mistakes is not easy, for most formal education is built on correct answers. Wrong answers are regarded as failures and are to be avoided. Parents conditioned to think this way are fostering an attitude that stands squarely in the way of encouraging children's self-direction and independence. People fearful of making mistakes will not risk trying. Without trying, self-direction, creativity, and independence cannot be discovered. One of the nice things about self-direction is that it does not have to be taught. It needs only to be encouraged.

Fourth, children with disabilities must learn the meaning of responsibility. The implications of decision-making experiences must be understood by them. Parenting should not be thought of as providing children with the correct answers but rather as providing them with opportunities to learn many ways of solving problems—not imaginary, make-believe problems but real ones in which decisions count.

RELIEVING PRESSURES

Wherever one goes in the world, one hears talk about external pressures that affect adults who do not have disabilities. At the same time that these people complain about the pressures that bother them, they do not seem to be fully aware of the pressures on people with disabilities. Individuals with disabilities are pressured to behave in a socialized way: to be popular, to belong to a group, to achieve in school, to hold their own in a competitive world, to take advantage of all opportunities, and to be happy in a world that even people without disabilities do not believe is safe and secure. In short, frequently, people with disabilities are expected to be better citizens than people without disabilities.

Children—with or without disabilities—cannot escape from all pressures, and it is not desirable that they do. A certain amount of pressure acts as a driving force, kindling the desire to finish a job or task, to go on to the next step. However, there are differences between constructive and destructive pressure. Constructive pressure is closely tied to two other parts of learning: motivation and the reward or satisfaction obtained through achievement. When conditions are not favorable for success and achievement, increased pressure is likely to result only in attitudes of distress and defeat. If parents are to aid their children in learning to live successfully with external pressures, they must know when to exert pressure.

Pressure applied for its own sake or a perverted reason ("to make them tough") will almost always fail, and parents who nag children to do better—without understanding why they are not making progress—will end up producing even greater underachievers. Pressure is positive only when it is combined with cues that arouse curiosity and interest and cause a person to exert pressure from within himself or herself to succeed. Parental pressure is of little value when the inner drive is missing in a child. Furthermore, success related to inner pressure is much more effective and infinitely more rewarding. Here, again, parents must be sure that pressure is applied toward a goal that is possible for a child to achieve. Negative pressure is often used carelessly by parents. A look of disappointment, sarcastic and undermining remarks, and comparing low-achieving children with siblings and peers are examples of negative pressures applied to shame a child into doing better. Such pressure tends to destroy children's faith in themselves as well as in their parents.

Obviously, if parents want their children to be optimally creative, external pressure is not the answer. Creativity develops from internal pressure. It comes from the reservoir of ideas that flow out of the mind and demand recognition. Parents can create an atmosphere or a safe place in which this can happen, but they cannot create the ideas. Children who feel comfortable at home — who find it safe to ask questions, express ideas, and try new behavior — respond to pressure within themselves through self-expression. They become well-balanced persons.

MARITAL PROBLEMS

When there is conflict centering on children, it is not helpful for parents to pretend that no conflict exists. Only by acknowledging that they have problems are they able to resolve them. Setting aside time to discuss points of distress is a good beginning, but it is only a beginning. Problem resolution must follow. Most parents forget that they were husbands and wives or lovers before they became parents. Ideally, they were even friends before becoming parents. They will need to build on all of these previous foundations to keep their marriage together. If the marriage is to survive, the neglected person must be brought back into the relationship.

Problem solving or adjusting to conflicts centering on a child with a disability can be one of the most trying aspects of a marriage. Running away from the issue by leaving home is not helpful. Another counterproductive approach is anger. However, productive anger is not the same as outbursts of hostility used exploitatively to get a spouse or a child to yield because of fear. Aristotle observed, "Anybody can become angry — that is easy; but to be angry with the right person, and to the right degree, and at the right time, and for the right purpose, and in the right way —

that is not within everybody's power and is not easy."

When conflicts arise and anger is one of the resulting emotions, the nonangry partner should realize that the anger is an indication of how strongly the other person feels about the situation. In this respect, feelings are emotional barometers that should be carefully read in order to predict the human relations climate. Often, there is a calm period before an outburst of anger. Silent suffering is seldom productive, particularly when the issue is a disabled child. If grievances are held in, tension will build up and eventually explode outward against the other partner or the child, or it will explode inward against the angry person and cause considerable psychological damage.

An important role for both partners in a marriage is listener. If one partner is troubled, the other needs to understand, and this requires listening. However, the listener should heed the words of the prophet Kahlil Gibran (1961): "The reality of the other person is not in what he reveals to you, but in what he cannot reveal to you. Therefore, if you would understand him, listen not to what he says but rather to what he does not say" (p. 14).* A major aspect of listening is being able to understand nonverbal messages—frowns, sighs, closed body positions.

Mothers in particular should make an attempt to include fathers in the care of the children. Fathers can feel abandoned, too. Most fathers want very much to be partners in nurturing and caring for their children. Love that grows in a family is best maintained by attachment and release. Attachment is in the form of closeness, companionship, and caring for each other, while release is in the form of trusting, respecting, and allowing the other person enough private space. In the center of this matrix are the children. If parents cannot let go of their children, the family becomes an unhealthy place. These families should have the following sign, like the warning on cigarettes, posted on their doors: "Beware, this family is dangerous to the health of its members."

Not all marriages that have a child with a disability turn sour, but many become emotionally colder. The disability is but another factor added to already strained interpersonal relations. As

---

*From Kahlil Gibran, *Sand and Foam*, 1961. Courtesy of Alfred A. Knopf, New York.

most marriages progress, disengagement tends to be the rule rather than the exception. Couples begin to pay less attention to each other; they frequently become bored with each other. The child with a disability is seldom the reason for the drifting apart, but he or she is often cited as the reason. Effective ways of coping can seldom be taught. At best, general guides can be offered, but each person must learn the coping styles that work in his or her situation. Drawing on the experiences of others gives parents a much-needed awareness that they are not the only ones with a particular problem but that, if they are not careful, they may be the only ones unable to resolve the problem. Help for children with disabilities must necessarily come from a network of persons— the children themselves, their parents, relatives, and friends, and professional and paraprofessional helpers.

ON CARING

In 1971, Milton Mayeroff wrote an insightful little book entitled *On Caring*. Little in the book is new, but Mayeroff's careful and warm way of restating old concepts pointed out the crucial role that caring plays in any sustaining human relationship. Parents of a child with a disability almost always say that they care *for* their child. Initially, most parents seem unable to care *about* their child. They care about their own thwarted dreams, but seldom do they care about the child who thwarts their dreams. Of course, there are other reasons—public embarrassment, shame, guilt, and other reaction that have been discussed—that make it easy to blame the child.

The lessons of the heart are infinitely more precious than the lessons of the head, but few parents of a child with a disability listen to their hearts. Instead, they treat their child like a book to be read, interpreted, and even marked on. Moreover, as they do with such a book, when the child becomes uninteresting or difficult to understand, parents give him or her away or throw him or her away. Sometimes a child with a disability becomes "the enemy" in the family—someone to be conquered, locked away, and guarded. In other families, a child with a disability becomes a pitiful person that parents and relatives call "poor baby." In rare, beautiful instances, children with disabilities are cared for and about as persons.

Parents who care about their children view them as being a part of themselves and also separate entities. They do not try to dominate or possess their children. Rather, they recognize their own and their children's need to grow. In order to do this, parents must feel good about themselves and their children. Self-honesty will allow parents to evaluate accurately their behavior and that of their children. No one would try to teach a turtle to fly or an elephant to bake a cake, but there are many things that turtles and elephants can do. Children are like turtles and elephants. Why try to teach blind children to pole-vault or deaf children to judge musical contests? There are many other things they can do. Caring parents have a true appreciation of their own potential abilities as well as their children's.

Caring is not a spectator sport; it requires active participation by all the parties involved. Parents who care learn from their mistakes and try not to repeat them. By modeling this behavior, they teach their children to learn from their mistakes, and in the process of learning, they develop humility. Parents learn from children, children learn from parents, and parents and children learn from themselves about themselves. They are not humiliated by having others see their weaknesses, nor are they vain when others see their strengths, for what they show is neither good nor bad. It is merely a condition that can be accepted or rejected. That is, they are never ashamed of themselves—of their negative behavior, perhaps, but never of themselves. Also, parents who care do not ask, "Aren't you ashamed of yourself?"

Parents who care about their children have a sense of humor. They are able to laugh at themselves and with their children. Kathryn Christenson and Kelvin Miller (1980) show how this is done. Humor is the lubricant that gets most parents over difficult spots, but they do not use humor to put down their children or to keep them dependent. Besides, as the saying goes, "Sometimes we laugh to keep from crying." There is something very funny about trying to be a superparent or superchild with a disability: None of them can fly, but all of them pretend to do so.

Parents who care about their child with a disability have a large amount of empathy and little sympathy. They do not hold out false hope to themselves or their child. Quick-fix solutions are not their style, and pity is buried in the past. These parents are realists. They talk with professionals who can help them to understand their child's diagnosis, treatment, and prognosis. They leave little to their fantasies and fears as they seek a clear prognosis and a clear understanding of the rehabilitation regimen. This is supplemented by current information about disabilities that is found in professional journals, textbooks, novels, autobiographies, and other library data. Caring parents tend to be well read.

Parents who care do not treat their children like the other-directed people David Reisman (1950) wrote about. Other-directed people are unable to distinguish thoughts from feelings and unable to express feelings even when recognizing them. Indeed, overprotected and overindulged children are unable to distinguish between what they want and what they ought to want. They become generally helpless, passive, and indecisive and have low self-esteem. Sadly, they defer to "normal" people when decisions about them are being made. It takes a lot of negative conditioning to produce other-directed people.

Parents who care meet their own physical and emotional needs. Individuals who give almost everything to others and little to themselves burn out as parents. Thus, they contribute to their own demise and that of their family. A truly caring relationship is mutually beneficial and, therefore, mutually growth producing and freeing. It is this freeing process that cements the bond that binds family members to one another. The binding is not in titles or ranks or physical conditions but in human beings caught up in each others' lives and yet free to let go if that will enrich them.

BURNOUT

The longer parents are together, the less they tend to do things together. Slowly a light seems to go out in their eyes, and they have difficulty seeing each other. The deadening effect of routine role conformity by parents of a child with a disability and the draining effects of trying to hide their feelings of frustration, loneliness, anger, and inadequacy should not be minimized. The inability of many individuals to find a way to relieve the incipient stress of parenting leads to *burnout*, the syndrome of emotional exhaustion and cynicism that occurs after long hours of physical and psychological strain. (This pertains not only to parents but to teachers and other human services personnel as well.)

In some cases, to burn out means that a parent will become an alcoholic, a drug addict, or mentally ill or even commit suicide. Herbert Freudenberger (1980) poetically and cogently summarized this decline: "Under the strain of living in our complex world, people's inner resources are consumed as if by fire, leaving a great emptiness inside, although the outer shells may be more or less unchanged" (p. xv). Contrary to many of their wishes or fantasies, parents are but mortal beings. Yet, there are numerous examples of parents who believe that they must be in control of themselves and their children at all times. Their children, they concede, can be out of control, but not them.

Some parents even believe that assisting their children to self-actualize is enough reward to keep themselves going. These martyrs get a kind of vicarious gratification from the successes of their children. Obviously this places a tremendous strain on their children to be socially successful. The self-denial of parents who push their own needs into the background is the volatile fuel that, when ignited, burns up their energies and dreams. There is a tendency for most parents to minimize the importance of self-love. Only if they have strong positive feelings for themselves are parents able to have these feelings for their children. However, parents who gratify their own appetite and emotions in self-destructive ways lack the qualities necessary to show their children restraint. It is a delicate balance that must be kept between self-love and self-indulgence.

It is erroneous to assume that burnout will disappear if it is ignored. This is a tragic belief because burnout does not get better by being ignored. The person burning out may be irritable, angry, resistant to change, or listless. Fatigue is a frequent symptom that many parents of a child with a disability experience because of the painful erosion of their ability to cope with their child's condition. Social symptoms include: (1) high resistance to going home, (2) a feeling of failure, (3) guilt and blame, (4) avoiding contact with friends, (5) reverting to strict rules and regulations, and (6) looking forward to the disabled child's going to sleep or away from home. Physical reactions to psychological stress centering on disabled children include: (1) migraine headaches, (2) backaches, (3) colds, (4) diarrhea, (5) excessive salivation or dryness of the mouth, (6) heartburn, (7) ulcers, (8) asthma, and (9) rhinitis. Sometimes parents can indeed acquire disabilities while trying to take care of their children. Moreover, burnout affects not just the isolated individual but the whole family.

Unlike romanticized television and movie programs, caring for children with disabilities is a tedious, unglamorous job. One should not dismiss too quickly the "burden" that many parents carry. Parents who burn out imagine themselves as somehow being responsible for the decisions and behaviors of their children. Thus, anguish, abandonment, and despair are natural responses to this unrealistic responsibility.

Most parents who accept this type of responsibility cannot help but feel a profound sense of guilt, even anxiety, when they choose destinies for their children. "Who can then prove that I am the proper person to impose, by my own choice, my conception of man upon mankind?" Jean-Paul Sartre (1965) asked. "If a voice speaks to me, it is still I myself who must decide whether the voice is or is not that of an angel" (p. 293). Burnout is sometimes the result of parents finding out that they hear neither angels nor devils, only human voices telling them what to do.

There are several ways parents can avoid burnout. Most parents do not do enough for themselves. Prolonged stress centering on a disabled child can affect the parents' personal lives away from home. It can make them unhappy with their loved ones and unable to be happy during "free" times and leave them generally listless and angry. Parents must learn to pay attention to physical symptoms, to put parenting goals in proper perspective, and to understand the nature of burnout. Only then can they control parenting activities rather than allowing the activities to control them. When parenting becomes a job, those who work at it must learn to vary it, leave it at times, and share it.

There are two reliable cures for burnout: closeness and being inner-directed. Closeness is anywhere and with anyone a person chooses. Before a person can achieve closeness with others, however, he or she has to achieve it with self. Parents who burn out seldom spend enough time with themselves in a constructive manner. Inner-directedness is not being selfish; rather, it is taking time out for oneself. The purpose, of course, is to do things that are good for one's renewal.

Parents should watch for tiredness and pay attention to physical symptoms such as colds or nagging pains in the back. Also, they should monitor themselves for shifts in attitude, especially toward self-doubt or self-pity. There are many other things parents can do to prevent burnout, including the following. Parents should (1) learn to ask for help, (2) be aware of their strengths and weaknesses, (3) take time out to do things they want to do, (4) learn to say no, (5) not feel guilty because they have not lived up to their ideal of a perfect parent, (6) exercise, and (7) set realistic goals for themselves. In order to help their children, parents must be good to themselves.

SUMMARY

The home is the key institution in personality formation. Children with disabilities have close ties with their parents in particular and other family members in general. Even in homes in which parents love and respect their children, there will be conflicts. Reacting to pressures in their own lives, some parents become demanding or overindulgent or overprotective. At the other end of the continuum, some parents abuse and neglect their children. Most parents manage to do a good job caring for themselves and their children. They would do a better job if they learned basic coping skills.

NOTE TO HELPERS

Parents and other family members vary in their ability to cope with disabilities. Professional helpers can assist them by providing them with needed information and, when appropriate, assurance that their feelings and emotions are part of the rehabilitation process. Deborah Kaplan and Judith Mearig (1977) suggested that informal problem solving is the most effective way professionals can help. This is not inconsistent with the goals of counseling, which include helping clients to become independent as soon as possible. Helpers should not expect instant coping or independence, however.

It is important that helpers do not try to rescue the family and make decisions for them, nor should they compete with parents and other family members for the affection of the child with a disability. Admittedly, it is difficult to care for the family instead of just the child, but this is exactly what the helper must do. The more effective treatment plans change to reflect changing family relationships. Failure to integrate rehabilitation goals and family members is likely to result in additional family stress and conflicts.

Most families have feelings of grief, hostility, guilt, and shame. They should not be made to feel guilty about their real and imagined inadequacies. It is unrealistic to expect them to handle their emotions and problems without help. Above all else, they need help understanding their feelings, the disability, and the treatment plan. Hilda Versluys (1980) offered a practical approach to helping the family adjust to the disability. Some of her suggestions are listed below.

- Be available and therapeutic with the family.
- Identify and appreciate the feelings of family members.
- Encourage and unconditionally accept ventilation of "hidden" feelings.
- Help family members see that their feelings are normal and acceptable.
- Keep the focus on real issues or crises.
- Provide praise for small accomplishments.
- Provide programs and services that are responsive to family and client needs.
- Discuss meaningful alternatives to rehabilitation problems.
- Provide information concerning procedures, simple facts about the disability, and purpose of treatment methods.
- Listen without offering false hope.

The helper must be able to project to the family an image of genuine concern, empathy, and technical skill. Even this may not be sufficient to dissolve family members' fears and anxieties, but it is a good place to begin. There is something inherently humbling about having a loved one with a physical or mental disability. Most frequently, family members take their cues from professional helpers. They need time to understand the disability and to learn how to cope with it. This is especially difficult when family members have not spent much time communicating about nondisability issues.

REFERENCES

Buscaglia, Leo. *The Disabled and Their Parents: A Counseling Challenge.* Thorofare, NJ: Charles B. Slack, 1975.

Christenson, Kathryn, and Miller, Kelvin. *Tributes to Courage.* Golden Valley, MN: Courage Center, 1980.

Featherstone, Helen. *A Difference in the Family: Life with a Disabled Child.* New York: Basic Books, 1980.

Freudenberger, Herbert J. *Burn-Out: The High Cost of Achievement.* New York: Doubleday, 1980.

Gibran, Kahlil. *Sand and Foam.* New York: Alfred A. Knopf, 1961.

Kaplan, Deborah, and Mearig, Judith S. A community support system for a family coping with chronic illness. *Rehab Lit, 38:* 79–82, 96, 1977.

Katz, Alfred H. *Parents of the Handicapped: Self-Organized Parents' and Relatives' Group for Treatment of Ill and Handicapped Children.* Springfield, IL: Charles C Thomas, 1961.

Kvaraceus, William C., and Hayes, E. Nelson (Eds.). *If Your Child Is Handicapped.* Boston: Porter Sargent, 1969.

Lewis, C. S. Quoted in Rosewell, Nelson. *Successful Living Day by Day.* New York: Macmillan, 1972.

Mayeroff, Milton. *On Caring.* New York: Harper & Row, 1971.

Perske, Robert. *Hope for the Families.* Nashville, TN: Abingdon, 1981.

Reisman, David. *The Lonely Crowd: A Study of the Changing American Character.* New Haven, CT: Yale University Press, 1950.

Ross, Bette M. *Our Special Child: A Guide to Successful Parenting of Handicapped Children.* New York: Walker, 1981.

Sartre, Jean-Paul. Quoted in Kaufman, Walter A. (Ed.). *Existentialism from Dosteovsky to Sartre.* New York: Meridan Books, 1965.

Spock, Benjamin M., and Lerrigo, Marion O. *Caring for Your Disabled Child.* New York: Macmillan, 1965.

Versluys, Hilda P. Physical rehabilitation and family dynamics. *Rehab Lit, 41:* 58–65, 1980.

Additional Readings

Abidon, Richard R. *Parenting Skills Workbook.* New York: Human Sciences Press, 1976.

Averbach, Stevanne. *The Whole Child: A Sourcebook.* New York: G. P. Putnam, 1981.

Benson, Leonard G. *Fatherhood: A Sociological Perspective.* New York: Random House, 1968.

Bigner, Jerry J. *Parent-Child Relations: An Introduction to Parenting.* New York: Macmillan, 1979.

Davis, Carroll. *Room to Grow: A Study of Parent-Child Relationships.* Toronto: University of Toronto Press, 1966.

Dunn, Judy. *Siblings: Love, Envy and Understanding.* Cambridge, MA: Harvard University Press, 1982.

Fraiberg, Selma H. *Every Child's Birthright: In Defense of Mothering.* New York: Basic Books, 1977.

Gordon, Thomas. *P. E. T., Parent Effectiveness Training.* New York: P. H. Wyden, 1970.

Goscrewski, F. William. *Effective Child Rearing: The Behaviorally Aware Parent.* New York: Human Sciences Press, 1976.

Mopsik, Stanley I., and Agard, Judith A. (Eds.). *An Education Handbook for Parents of Handicapped Children.* Cambridge, MA: Abt Books, 1980.

Power, Paul W., and Dell Orto, Arthur E. *Role of the Family in the Rehabilitation of the Physically Disabled.* Baltimore: University Park Press, 1980.

Rosenblatt, Gary C. *Parental Expectations and Attitudes about Childbearing in High-Risk vs. Low-Risk Child-Abusing Families.* Saratoga, CA: Century Twenty One, 1980.

Satir, Virginia M. *Peoplemaking.* Palo Alto, CA: Science and Behavior Books, 1972.

Teele, James E. *Mastering Stress in Child Rearing: A Longitudinal Study of Coping.* Lexington, MA: Lexington Books, 1981.

Chapter 9

TIPS FOR TEACHERS

How people with disabilities are taught matters as much as what they are taught. Teachers should carefully decide how they can best help each needy student. For, indeed, teachers are *guides* who show students the pathways to acquiring an education. As guides, they determine the pace and sequence of the trip; they decide which routes should be taken; it is their responsibility to make the journey interesting and informative for the student traveler. The teacher guides, with their zest for the subject, must awaken a desire in their students and instill within them the tenacity to complete the journey.

Teachers are *models* for their students, an example that the children can follow. This is one of the greatest responsibilities of teachers and one from which few educators can escape. Good or bad, teachers are role models. This part of education is enhanced when teachers gain insight, understanding, and friendship with students of all groups. The impressions teachers make remain forever in the minds of students.

Teacher as *counselors* bear great responsibility for advising students. Students with disabilities are continually faced with problems and decisions related to their disabilities. During times of extreme stress, most students turn to their teachers for guidance. In this capacity, teachers are able to bend and shape persons with disabilities toward many forms of behavior that carry over to subsequent nonschool activities. Insensitive educators fail during these periods, and in so doing they cause students to fail. When given an opportunity to offer advice, it is important that teachers do not belittle this role.

Teachers are *actors*. Being effective in the classroom is much like being effective on the stage of a theater or in a movie. What often seems like a natural performance is the result of much hard work. An actor reads over a script, decides he likes it, and studies it until he knows it. When he is competent, he goes on the stage and portrays his character so that it communicates with the members of the audience and they come to know the content of the character before they leave the theater. It is much the same with effective teachers. They come across an aspect of teaching they like, go to college, and study that area until they know it. Then they go into the community and present their educational knowledge to students. Before the performance ends, the students come to know the teachers as either good or bad.

For students with disabilities, the chief work of teachers is helping them learn how to learn. This means helping them to define their interests, needs, and abilities; helping them to understand themselves better; and otherwise helping them to become wise consumers and useful citizens. Basic to being an effective teacher is knowing oneself. Arthur Jersild (1953) succintly pointed out: "One can master the facts, principles, and laws contained in a hundred books on psychology and still understand neither oneself nor others. Self-understanding requires integrity rather than mere cleverness. It involves emotion. To know oneself, one must be able to recognize feelings, act them, and deal with them in constructive ways; and this is something quite different from reading or talking about them with detachment" (p. 9).

THE HELPING PROCESS

All definitions of teaching are based on subjective values, something tangible or intangible discovered in a relationship between a teacher and a student. In actuality, help in the teaching process is only offered; it cannot be given. Each student must accept or reject information offered by the teacher. The ultimate responsibility for learning belongs to the student.

Some teachers see the helping process as one in which they make intricate diagnoses of the learning abilities and personal lives of students and then use a wide variety of instructional techniques with them. Still other teachers see students with disabilities as being suitable for living only in sheltered environments.

The relationships of these teachers with students are not really helping relationships. On the contrary, they are controlling relationships. When students with disabilities become objects of pity rather than of learning, they are no longer persons who act but instead become things manipulated.

Martin Buber (1958) described manipulation in terms of an I-It relationship, the opposite to the loving I-Thou relationship. I-It relationships are dehumanizing and destructive. They can lead to error because they create a false picture of who one is in the universal system. If one is the I, this causes one to define oneself as superior to all others, and with such a perception it is impossible to enter into mutual relations with others. People with disabilities, when seen as the Its in relationships of this nature, cease to be people and become the equivalent of wheelchairs, canes, hearing aids, and braces.

There is an underlying assumption in the teaching profession that college-trained persons can make a significant positive contribution to the lives of students if their training has instilled commitment to use themselves effectively in the helping process. Clearly, the primary technique or instrument in teacher-student relationships is the ability of the teacher to become an instrument to be used by all students to achieve *their* educational goals. From the teacher's point of view, fulfillment of this goal means that the students will become more realistic and self-directing.

Certain values in teacher-student relationships must be observed by teachers if all students are to be productive in the long run. Doing a chore or making a decision for students with disabilities may help in the short run, but it will not help them to become more self-directing and knowledgeable about life decisions in the future. In their desire to do everything for their students, many teachers enslave them; the students become academic cripples who believe that their teachers are the only ones who can decide for them and do not learn to take care of themselves. Some helpful teacher beliefs are as follows:

1. The belief that human life, happiness, and well-being are to be valued above all else.
2. The belief that students with disabilities should be given an

opportunity to be the masters of their lives, with the right to
control them in their own interests and in their own ways, as
long as the exercise of this control does not infringe on the
rights of other people.

3. The belief that the dignity and worth of each student shall be
respected at all times.
4. The belief in the right of all students to think their own
thoughts and speak their own minds.

It is a teacher's basic beliefs and values rather than his or her
grand schemes, methods, or techniques that are the real determiners of students' classroom adjustment. Specifically related to
teaching students with disabilities, the major task of the teacher is
to provide classroom experiences in which realistic choices are
possible. Ideally, through teacher-student interactions the fears
and anxieties that restrain students can to some extent be resolved,
and they can make a commitment to a course of action and learn
how to make their decisions a reality. Of course, there will be
instances when students do not achieve their goals, i.e. when the
goals are too difficult, when students lack the motivation to learn,
or when they are conditioned to fail. If skillfully handled, however,
these instances are not perceived by the students as personal
failures. Rather, they are identified as situations in which they can
learn how to cope with barriers to specific educational goals.

In a classic article entitled "The Characteristics of a Helping
Relationship," Carl Rogers (1958) asked a series of questions that
he felt revealed characteristics of a helping relationship. If teachers
can answer these questions in the affirmative, especially concerning most of their interactions with students who have disabilities,
then it is likely that they will be or are helpful to all their students.

- *Can I be in some way which will be perceived by the other person as
trustworthy, as dependable or consistent in some deep sense?*

  This is more than being rigidly consistent. It means being
  honest and congruent with feelings to be a unified or an
  integrated person. If teachers cannot work with certain students,
  they should refer them to someone who they think can.

- *Can I be expressive enough as a person that what I am will be
communicated unambiguously?*

If teachers are unaware of their own feelings, they will send a double message that will confuse the situation and cause the student-teacher relationship to be marred by the ambiguous communication.

• *Can I let myself experience positive attitudes toward this other person — attitudes of warmth, caring, liking, interest, respect?*
An attitude of aloofness is unhelpful; it creates a barrier or distance that projects scientific objectivity at the expense of establishing a professional relationship.

• *Can I receive him as he is? Can I communicate this attitude? Or can I only receive him conditionally, acceptant of some aspects of his feelings and silently or openly disapproving of other aspects?*
Teachers usually are threatened when they cannot accept certain parts of their students' behavior or personality. To be helpful, teachers must be able to accept even those personality characteristics of students that they would not adopt — that is, as long as these characteristics do not harm others. Again, teachers should refer students to someone else if they feel unable to accept them.

• *Can I act with sufficient sensitivity in the relationship that my behavior will not be perceived as a threat?*
If students with disabilities are as free as possible from external threats, then they are better able to experience and to deal with the internal feelings pertaining to their disabilities, which are threatening.

• *Can I let myself enter fully into the world of his feelings and personal meanings and see these as he does? Can I step into his private world so completely that I lose all desire to evaluate or judge it? Can I enter it so sensitively that I can move about it freely, without trampling on meanings which are precious to him? Can I sense it so accurately that I can catch the meanings which are implicit, which he sees only dimly or as confusion? Can I extend this understanding without limit?*
Evaluative comments are not conducive to personal growth, and therefore they should not be a part of teacher-student relationships. For example, positive evaluation ("I agree") is threatening because it serves notice that the student is being evaluated and a negative evaluation ("I disagree") could be

forthcoming. Self-evaluation ("What do you think?") leaves the responsibility where it really belongs—with the students. In essence, the ultimate question becomes,

- *Can I meet disabled students as persons who are in the process of becoming, or will I be bound by their disabilities and my biases?*
This question gets to the heart of learning barriers related to physical disabilities.

Four subtle attitudinal characteristics are necessary for optimum teacher-student interactions to occur: (1) Teachers must manifest *empathic understanding* of their students; (2) teachers must manifest *unconditional positive regard* toward their students; (3) teachers must be *genuine* or *congruent;* that is, their words match their feelings; and (4) the teachers' responses must match the students' statements in intensity of affective expression. Of course, these four conditions must be communicated to students. In an effort to conceptualize this process, Rogers (1961) formulated what he calls a *process equation* of a successful helping relationship: Genuineness plus empathy plus unconditional positive regard for the student equals successful interaction (G + E + UPR = Success).

Verbally, teachers can convey genuineness, empathy, and unconditional positive regard to students with disabilities through four statements and the feelings and actions that accompany them: "This is the way it is." "I know that some aspects of this may be difficult." "I am here to help you if you want me and can use me." "You don't have to face this alone." These statements contain reality, empathy, and support or acceptance. The words of these statements are only one part of the communication process, however. Appropriate action must follow. As an old Indian once said about the treatment his people received from whites, "What you do speaks so loudly I cannot hear what you say!"

To be effective, reality *and* empathy must be conveyed to students with disabilities. As Alan Keith-Lucas (1972) wrote: "Reality without empathy is harsh and unhelpful. Empathy about something that is not real is clearly meaningless and can only lead the client to what we have called non-choice. Reality and empathy together need support, both material and psychological, if decisions are to be carried out. Support in carrying out unreal plans is obviously a waste of time" (p. 88).

Many studies that focus on the nature of helping in the classroom support the ideas of Rogers and others and indicate that three recurring behaviors are relevant to people who are considering entering the teaching profession:

1. The teacher's ability sensitively and accurately to perceive all students in such a manner as to communicate deep understanding

2. The teacher's ability to project nonpossessive warmth and acceptance of students

3. The necessity for the teacher to be integrated, mature, and genuine within the relationship

Three characteristics of a successful helping relationship—genuineness, empathy, and acceptance—that seem vital to the teaching profession will be examined next.

Genuineness

Lowell wrote, "Sincerity is impossible unless it pervades the whole being, and the pretense of it saps the very foundation of character." To be genuine in teacher-student relationships requires teachers to be aware of their own inner feelings. If their feelings are consistent with their expressed behavior, then it can be said that teachers are *genuine* and *congruent.* This the quality of realness and honesty allows students needing help to keep a steady focus on reality. To the squeamish teacher, it may seem that reality is too brutal for persons with disabilities. Granted, the truth is not always painless; as the old saying goes, "The truth shall make ye free—but first it shall make ye miserable." It also is important to note that being open and honest is not a license to be brutal. Helpful as opposed to destructive comments are very much like the differences between a fatal and a therapeutic dose of a painkiller—a matter of degree.

In the process of attempting to be transparently real, it is wise for teachers to evaluate their reasons for being less than honest. To protect students with disabilities from the truth about themselves is to say that they are incapable of facing their real problems. It is vitally important for each student to be aware of his or her educational development. However, if teachers provided only honesty in the relationship, it probably would not be very helpful. The next component in the teaching process, empathic understanding, is needed also.

Empathy

"First of all," he said, "if you can learn a simple trick, Scout, you'll get along a lot better with all kinds of folks. You never really understand a person until you consider things from his point of view—"
"Sir?"
"—until you climb into his skin and walk around in it."
[Lee, 1960, p. 36*]

This passage from *To Kill a Mockingbird* accurately depicts the meaning of *empathic understanding*. It is literally an understanding of the emotions and feelings of another, not by the cognitive process but by a projection of one's personality into the personality of the other. It is a sort of vicarious experiencing of the feelings of the other: Teachers actually feel some of the emotions of students. Empathy requires teachers to leave their own lifespaces temporarily and to try to think, act, and feel as if the life spaces of persons with disabilities were their own. No one can ever feel *like* other persons but should be able to feel *with* them.

It is important that teachers maintain enough objectivity in their empathy so that they can assist students with disabilities to overcome problems related to their disabilities. Neither teachers nor students should wallow in pity. Also, empathic understanding does no good unless it is communicated to students. It is comforting to them to know that someone has a deep understanding of their predicament. This kind of understanding allows students to expand and clarify their own self-understanding. One way of communicating understanding is through *active listening*, which is not mere tolerance. Teachers, for instance, have to really care and feel the emotions attached to students' words. The following four points express what *listening with empathic understanding* means.

1. It means trying to see the situation the way the other person sees it.

---

*From *To Kill a Mockingbird* by Harper Lee (J. B. Lippincott Co.). Copyright © 1960 by Harper Lee. Reprinted by permission of Harper & Row, Publishers, Inc.

2. It means entering actively and imaginatively into the other person's situation and trying to understand a frame of reference different from one's own.

3. It does not mean maintaining a polite silence while one rehearses what one is going to say when given a chance.

4. It does not mean waiting alertly for the flaws in the other person's argument so that one can correct him or her.

Once teachers are behaving genuinely and have empathic understanding toward students with disabilities, the next step, which often occurs simultaneously, is accepting.

Acceptance

Acceptance of students with disabilities means that teachers feel and show unconditional positive regard for them. Teachers must be congruent or consistent in both their feelings and their expressions of acceptance for disabled students. If teachers do not really accept students but attempt to express acceptance, they give a double message: acceptance and rejection. In such a case, the best that can happen is that the students perceive these individuals to be phonies. The worst that can happen is that the students' self-esteem is damaged.

Double messages occur when feelings do not coincide with words. For instance, a teacher's words may say, "I accept you and respect your feelings," but the nonverbal message may say, "Don't touch me, you are ugly." Nonverbal messages are difficult to correct because one does not have as much control over them as over words. Most people intuitively know this and are perceptive enough to sense the feelings. The words of Joe Louis to one of his boxing opponents summarize this point: "You can run but you can't hide from me."

The major reasons for demonstrating acceptance are to build a relationship based on trust and openness, to establish a situation in which all members of the class are able to gain additional respect for themselves, and to develop an atmosphere through which the students can respect their teacher. The basic process involved in this aspect of the relationship is *caring*, and support is given through helpful feedback. *Feedback* is simply the expression of reactions to a behavior. In a sense, students perceive the teacher's attitude of respect as an "either/or" thing: The teacher either does or does not respect them. This may be an oversimplification, but if students perceive in this manner, the consequences of that perception are real.

To the extent that teachers can be themselves as persons, expressing their real selves, they will have empathic understanding for their students, but teachers are not social workers, physicians, or psychiatrists. They should dispense course materials, not therapy. In searching for the helping relationship in teaching, it would be wise to remember the following Zen poem:

> It is too clear and so hard to see.
> A man once searched for fire with a lighted lantern.
> Had he known what fire was,
> He could have cooked his rice much sooner.

THE FIRST TEACHER-STUDENT CONTACT

Only as teachers study and practice do they become proficient in their profession. There are many special education courses that sensitize neophytes to methods for effectively teaching students with disabilities. However, while in college, the student teacher does not learn how to teach but rather about teaching. During this period, most students come to understand the meaning of the phrase, "A prerequisite to learning is a good attitude." Teachers must feel good about themselves and feel good about being teachers before they can become effective in the classroom. Even though generalizations are hazardous, the following tips seem to apply to teachers of all students. Teachers should—

1. attempt to understand the feelings of students and to empathize with them.
2. see students as worthy beings, even when disapproving of their behavior.
3. believe that all students are able to learn.
4. try to understand the classroom conditions that may negatively affect students but not stereotype them.
5. seek ways to reach and interest students.

6. set clear, fair rules for each class and be firm in holding to them.
7. accept differences in physical and cultural conditions as well as individual behaviors without showing signs of shock or ridiculing students.
8. recognize individual and variant styles of learning and try to adapt teaching methods to fit them.
9. identify and utilize the strengths in all students.
10. give students praise and concrete rewards and recognize the importance of each individual's experiencing success.

Frank Broadbent and Donald Cruickshank (1965) stated that most beginning teachers wish for a list of foolproof techniques for coping with classroom problems. Unfortunately, there are no lists of infallible rules for teachers, beginning or experienced, to follow. Therefore, each teacher must compile his or her own list. The teacher-student relationship is too personal to be reduced to a single formula, however. Indeed, the teacher-student relationship is more than an adult-child or boss-subordinate relationship. It is a human relationship at the most intimate level. Relatedly, there are fears that most teachers have concerning it.

Fear is one of the most troublesome of all emotional reactions. It is an overriding belief that some ominous danger threatens. Fear tends to unnerve one at a time when one most needs to be calm. Often the source of the fear is not known, has been forgotten, or is repressed. Sidney Jourard (1963) said that fear is a barrier to reality testing. It takes courage to face the truth, and frequently this courage is lacking. One's security and self-esteem are threatened when one becomes afraid. Gordon Allport (1958) compared fear to a grease spot that spreads throughout life and stains an individual's social relationships. Like aggression, most teachers are ashamed of fear since their ethical codes place a high premium on courage and self-reliance. Teachers who are anxious about teaching children with disabilities often imagine that they are surrounded by dangerous forces: defective equipment, uneducable students, and nonsupportive administrators. Some of these anxieties develop into phobias. Jesse Gordon (1963) wrote:

> Phobias are usually experienced as strong apprehension and anxiety when in the presence of the phobic object or situation, a fear that can

develop into panic proportions in which the person blindly flees in a loss of self-control from the phobic situation. Objects associated with the phobic object acquire the capacity to elicit the fear, through stimulus generalization. The phobic person usually takes steps to avoid the phobic situation, and these steps often produce a restriction on his life which makes it more difficult for him to engage in the usual social interactions. [P. 497]

In extreme cases, the mere thought of teaching certain students is enough to produce physiological states of anxiety, e.g. a rapid heart rate, upset stomach, sweating, and trembling. Mild anxiety improves the teaching performance, but high anxiety lowers it. Most teachers want their students to think highly of them, and they, in turn, want to think highly of their students. The likelihood of either condition occurring is slight if teachers have a phobia about students with disabilities.

It is typical for teachers to dread their first or a new assignment. This fear is not completely groundless. It is possible to progress through an entire teacher preparation program with a high prognosis of becoming a successful teacher only to be tripped up and disillusioned by unexpected classroom failures. Many teachers believe being assigned students who are "abnormal" will result in such an experience. Also, because students with disabilities are perceived as being physically weaker than other students, most teachers are unsure of how to discipline them. More than anything, this is fear of the unknown.

Discipline

Classroom control is a matter for each individual teacher to develop. What works well for one teacher may not ensure success for another. The same discipline administered by different teachers can have vastly dissimilar results. A teacher's fear of unruly students with physical disabilities is, for the most part, unfounded. The great majority of students with physical disabilities are not discipline problems. If they perceive their teachers to be fair, sincere persons, these students usually are quite receptive to their classroom programs and procedures. A major cause of the problems that many teachers experience is their inability to relate to students with an appreciable degree of human warmth. These teachers define students with disabilities as *animals* and themselves as *zookeepers*. Their foremost job, they believe, is to keep the animals quiet. Consequently, their classes are places of "No," "Quiet" and "Shut up." The students are to be seen but not heard. Ideally, they should not even be seen. Needless to say, teachers who do not care about students with disabilities find few positive things to say about them and are quick to punish them.

At the other end of the continuum, there are teachers who believe that the students' disabilities are enough punishment and, therefore, they do not need to be disciplined. In this situation, students with disabilities are not corrected for misdeeds that bring negative sanctions to other students. Teachers behaving this way rationalize that someone or something else is at fault, absolving the students of their guilt. This is not kindness, for as students grow and learn to live with their disabilities or to overcome them to some degree, the problem of discipline, especially self-discipline, becomes a greater problem or handicap than their physical disability.

There is a risk in disciplining students with disabilities. Teachers who do so may be viewed by their colleagues and friends as "mean" persons, probably the meanest on earth. To the insensitive onlookers, these teachers have no heart at all. However, these "heartless" teachers know that to let disabled students use their disabilities to gain special attention or to get special dispensations or special treatment is worse than the actual disabilities. People who lose an arm or leg can teach the remaining limbs to take over; the hard-of-hearing can learn to read lips and nonverbal cues; the blind can learn to "see" with their hands and ears. During these processes, people with disabilities should also learn to accept responsibility for their behaviors.

Although it is impossible to prepare a detailed and well-planned approach to every classroom situation and thereby guarantee student receptiveness, teachers can plan activities that will improve classroom interaction. It is known by the more effective educators that students with disabilities respond more favorably to teachers who utilize classroom techniques that demonstrate consistent conduct and procedures than they do to teachers whose techniques are inconsistent and unstable. They feel relaxed and secure when they are exposed to classrooms characterized by consistent teacher behavior. When students, with or without disabilities, cannot anticipate with a great degree of accuracy what their teachers will do, they feel insecure. Students who are subjected to classroom conditions and procedures that appear to be unsettled or unstable tend to panic and misbehave. Although teachers may not be able to develop a pattern of action that ensures total classroom control, they can control most aspects of the classroom interaction.

Students do not always act up because of social maladjustment. For instance, they may misbehave because they are physically ill. Some restless students have hyperthyroid conditions that need medical attention. In any case, effective classroom control requires an understanding of each student's social and physical conditions. Students who act up in class may be frustrated, angry, physically ill, or all three; seldom are they uncontrollable.

Personal Characteristics

It is difficult to convince new teachers that they probably will experience no major catastrophe in their initial assignments. Only actual experiences that bear this out are adequate reassurances. Sometimes, too, teachers have good reasons to be anxious about how students with disabilities will respond to them. In fact, they have good reasons to be anxious about how the other students will respond to them, also. This is because there may be something about them that triggers rejection. (Interestingly, many of the things that turn off students also irritate other teachers.) Specifically, young teachers or youthful-looking teachers may doubt their ability to control students who are very near their own age. In addition, new teachers often worry about their personality. Will it be compatible with those of the students?

Certainly, a new teacher should be concerned with all of the above considerations. Yet, it must be recognized that teachers differ from one another in size, weight, shape, degree of attractiveness, and personality development. The majority of students are not too concerned with how youthful a teacher looks, nor are they obsessed with any great preference for teachers who are beautiful by "normal" standards while others are less attractive. On the contrary, students with disabilities tend to be more concerned with the following questions:

1. Is the teacher able to put students at ease?

2. Is the teacher's approach to students positive?

3. Is the teacher able to present course material in an interesting and meaningful way?

4. Is the teacher sincere?

5. Does he or she have a sense of humor?

6. Does the teacher have a real concern for persons with disabilities?

Teachers should make every effort to understand the worlds of *all* students. This includes learning about their growth patterns, interests, and social codes. Gaps in understanding students almost always facilitate student failures. Conversely, the students' misunderstanding of their teachers also facilitates failure. The key to both situations is to seek understanding, not to assess blame. An old adage seems relevant, "There is so much good in the worst of us, and so much bad in the best of us, that it ill behooves any of us to find any fault with the rest of us."

It is not enough to stimulate students to learn. They must be involved in the learning process, in setting their goals and in evaluating their progress. Thus, students, even and perhaps especially students with disabilities, should be free to interact within their classes, which also involves assuming responsibility for their behavior. The self-esteem of these students is weakened by teachers who treat them like pets and fragile dolls but not people.

SOCIAL CLASS AND HELPERS

It may be helpful for teachers to be aware of some other aspects of helping. Specifically, most writers suggest that four things must occur before people ask for help:

1. They must recognize that something is wrong that they can do nothing about without help.

2. They must be willing to tell someone about their problem.

3. They must give that person the right to assist in analyzing their behavior.

4. They must be willing to change in some way.

All of this is very threatening to the equilibrium and self-concept of people with disabilities, who take pride in not asking for help. In this highly competitive society, lower-class students with disabilities are in a particularly difficult situation because of their relatively limited funds and high dependence on other people. To them, seeking help in school is viewed as yet another degrading process.

As to the actual kind of helping relationship established with students from the lower socioeconomic classes, male students from this group dislike talk and have a strong preference for action. In fact, males in most social classes tend to be more secretive than females and more afraid to talk about their inner feelings. Chapter 5 discussed this as an aspect of *machismo*. When there is difficulty in verbalizing feelings, silence is the loudest and most agonizing sound that teachers will hear. It is helpful to be patient and let students tell their story in their own way and at their own pace. In addition to feeling uncomfortable, lower-strata students generally are less verbal in the classroom. This does not mean that they are nonverbal, however.

Numerous studies have focused on the helping relationship as a function of social class and ethnicity. August Hollingshead and Frederick Redlich (1958) observed that therapists have more positive feelings toward clients whose social class is comparable to their own. It seems reasonable to speculate that most teachers, then, have more positive feelings for students having disabilities who are of their own socioeconomic class than for those of another. George Banks, Bernard Berenson, and Robert Carkhuff (1967) found that counselors who are different from their clients in terms of race and ethnic identity have the greatest difficulty effecting constructive changes, while counselors who are similar to their clients have the greatest facility for doing so. One could speculate that teachers of the same ethnic background as their students have the least difficulty establishing rapport with them. This does not mean that social class and ethnicity are insurmountable barriers, though.

It is important to note that students with disabilities need more (or a different kind of) attention than other students. Of course, this is an overgeneralization, since each student should be looked at individually in order to determine his or her personal needs. Even so, it is imperative that teachers be cognizant of barriers created by social class and physical differences. If students with disabilities are hesitant to trust a teacher, for example, it may be that they do not trust people in general, or it may be that the teacher's nonverbal messages say, "Stay away." Rather than guess, it is better to ask students what they think the difficulty may be. If done tactfully, this will get the issue out in the open with a minimum of defensiveness. It may be that the students are not aware of their own nontrusting behavior, or the teacher may have been projecting his or her own nontrusting attitude onto the students. In any case, it is best to get and keep these feelings, perceptions, and thoughts out in the open so that trust can be built.

This does not mean that helping relationships are always nice and sweet. The following interview by Alfred Benjamin (1969) tells of a helping relationship that a student had with a teacher that was not always pleasant.

> He was my teacher for three years in junior high school, and I gave him hell. I was a devil then and hated the guy. That's what I thought then, but it wasn't only hate. He didn't let me get away with a thing in class, and lots of times he'd keep me in after school to talk things over. He told me exactly how he felt, and I remember I told him lots of things. . . . I don't know why exactly. . . . I think, because I trusted him.
>
> Now that I think of it, that teacher never told me he was right and I was wrong. He said there were things I was doing he couldn't allow, or something like that, and he told me why. I told him how I felt about the kids in the class and how boring school was. He listened to it. We never got to see eye to eye on lots of things, but we knew where we stood. I know now that I learned more from him in those talks than I did during four years in high school. I didn't know it then, but he taught me to think and to see what I was doing. After a while he had enough, I guess, and I don't blame him. He gave me up for lost, I suppose, and he'll never know how much he helped me. It took me years to find it out. [Pp. 92–93]

Most problems that students have are rooted in their social environments. More laws is an alternative solution to these problems. Another alternative is action designed to change colleges of education. Neither of these, however, is the complete solution. One of the reasons many teachers are continually frustrated is that the problems they are called upon to solve are themselves the products of other institutions and community organizations. If teachers really want to be helpful, some of them will have to be active in community change. Usually, the most significant changes that they can make involve their own classroom behaviors.

Frequently the school adjustment of students with disabilities depends not on relocation in their present school but instead on being moved to another school. This kind of environmental change is not without precedent. It is modeled after milieu therapy and preventative and community or social psychiatry. However, more often than not, students with disabilities do not get the assistance they need because few schools are attuned to their needs. Six things teachers can and must do if students, with and without disabilities, are to be given the best possible education are:

1. Regard each student as an important member of the class.

2. View all students positively, because whatever diminishes a student's self—humiliation, degradation, or failure—has no place in the education profession.

3. Provide for individual differences; do not stereotype students because of their skin color, physical condition, income, or ethnic identity.

4. Apply empathy to every teaching experience.

5. Allow ample opportunities for all students to explore the learning experiences within their ability to participate.

6. Learn from mistakes and do not repeat them.

Because sensitivity to one's own feelings is a prerequisite to effective helping, it may be beneficial for teachers who have not done so to undergo some type of human relations training. Studies indicate that a large number of persons who teach students with disabilities are in need of some kind of top-quality experiential training. Other studies provide extensive evidence that teachers who have actively participated in such programs are more successful in helping students with disabilities. Yet, even with this training, teachers may fail because of the delicate nature of the caring relationship, which Thomas Gordon (1970) described in the following passage:

You and I are in a relationship with each other. Yet each of us is a separate person having his own needs. I will try to be as accepting as I can of your behavior. But I can be genuinely accepting of you only as long as your behavior to meet your needs does not conflict with my meeting my own needs. Therefore, whenever I am feeling nonaccepting of you because my own needs are not being met, I will tell you as openly and honestly as I can, leaving it up to you whether you will change your behavior. I also will encourage you to do the same with me and will try to listen to your feelings and perhaps change my behavior. However, when we discover that a conflict-of-needs continues to exist in our relationship, let us both commit ourselves to try to resolve that conflict without the use of either my power or yours. I will respect your needs, but I also must respect my own. Consequently, let us strive always to search mutually for solutions to our inevitable conflicts that will be acceptable to both of us. In this way, your needs will be met but so will mine. As a result, you can continue to grow and achieve satisfaction and so can I. And, finally, our relationship can continue to be a healthy one because it will be mutually satisfying. [Pp. 424–425]

EDUCATIONAL NEEDS OF STUDENTS WITH DISABILITIES

Much of the plight of students with disabilities stems from the inability of their teachers to understand them. Many teachers erroneously think that these students are alien people having needs unlike those of "normal" students. A closer analysis of their behavior shows that it is not the classroom adjustment patterns of students with disabilities that are "abnormal" but their opportunities to behave as "normal" students. All students have the following educational needs.

1. The Need Not to Be Loved to Death

Students with disabilities do not need misplaced kindness; instead they need empathic but fair guidance. Often teachers attempt to "make up" for disabilities by giving students unearned rewards. No matter how well intended, social promotions and watered-down assignments cause additional problems. With so much emphasis currently being placed on understanding and assisting students with disabilities, it is easy to fall victim to the urge to engage in overcompensatory actions. This may lead to the disabled student syndrome.

The *disabled student syndrome* refers to the process by which students with disabilities use their disabilities to beat the school system. "When I want to get out of doing my schoolwork," a high school student said, "I just lie and tell my teachers that my back hurts." This is beating the system — getting by without doing the required work. Using their physical disabilities as a crutch, some students with disabilities hobble through school, manipulating their perceived manipulators (school personnel). Few students in this category are seeking a top-quality education. They seek only to minimize the complications during their stay in school.

To students who know that they are not putting forth the required effort but receiving rewards and praise anyway, success in school is meaningless. Yet, using the old maxim that the shortest distance between two points is a straight line, these students are content to get through school by exerting minimal intellectual effort. School under these conditions becomes a game in which they lose even if they get high grades. Making it easy for students to succeed without doing minimum proficiency work also makes it easy for them to fail in the world of work. Students with disabilities need not less education than their peers but the same, not less challenge but the same.

2. The Need to Receive Consistent and Fair Evaluations

Too often, teachers assume that all or most students with physical disabilities are of low intelligence. Along with this assumption goes the belief that these students do not know the difference between properly executed and improperly executed school assignments. As a result, some teachers capriciously parcel out rewards and punishments. Unlike loving students to their academic deaths, teachers who treat the disabled this way are indifferently thwarting their desire to compete for school success symbols.

Negatively prepared for academic life, many students with disabilities desperately need meaningful evaluations to get them turned on to school. This means that they should be given not high grades or praise for low achievement but, instead, appropriate recognition for the work they do. It is easier for students to adjust to consistent than capricious teachers. "I don't mind him giving me a *D* for my score," an angry student said, "but he gave me a *C* for the same score last week." Feeling confused and powerless to do anything about it, these students give up and sink deeper into the mire of mediocrity. *Good work* and *bad work* become synonymous with *wasted work.* If enough teachers respond in this manner, students with disabilities do not drop out: They are pushed out.

3. *The Need to Be Accepted as Human Beings*

Students with disabilities need teachers who can touch, smell, and smile at them. Teachers who view them as being highly contagious disease germs subconsciously or consciously try to avoid contact with them. The best method for gaining the confidence of students with disabilities is not periodically reminding them verbally of acceptance but showing them through actions. Teachers who periodically give an "I understand your handicap" lecture are suspect. They are suspected of being insincere. In fact, when students test these teachers' sincerity, many of them, like the one who violently jumped back when a student with cerebral palsy tried to touch her, fail their moments of truth.

All students need to be accepted as worthy beings. The classroom cutup illustrates this point: While unable to gain recognition under calmer conditions, a student acting out in class may goad a reluctant teacher into touching him. Students with disabilities have the same educational needs as other students. That is, all students need teachers who will (1) be honest in evaluating their work, (2) tell them where they are in their subject development, and (3) assist them in their efforts to improve.

William James said, "An unlearned carpenter of my acquaintance once said in my hearing: 'There is very little difference between one man and another; but what little there is, is very important.'" The behavior of most students is good and desirable. A healthy student with a disability is a person who enjoys learning and is a joy to teach. *Health,* then, refers to classroom disposition and behavior. It has little to do with physical disability. As noted earlier, healthy students are free to make choices. They are free to sift through alternatives and choose the best ones. They do not use their disabilities as excuses for failures or reasons for success.

All people have options, and they make choices every day. Yet, not all choices are made out of awareness. An example of making an unaware choice is losing control of one's temper and blaming others for this loss, i.e. "You made me angry." An example of making a choice through awareness is the expression of direct anger, i.e. "I will not complete the assignment because the books present untrue discussions of disabled people." If anger is turned inward, it becomes depression. If it is turned outward without responsibility, it becomes hostility. If anger is expressed outwardly with responsibility and directly at the source of anger, the result is anger with awareness. Continuing the illustration used above, the student can complete the assignment but document the negative aspects of the books and recommend more appropriate ones.

The healthy student with a disability is a self-regulated person. Self-regulation is learned early in life and continues to strengthen and develop as the individual matures. Self-regulation means the right to live freely, without undue outside authority. Healthy students operate in the here and now. They are primarily concerned with the present, not the past. They do not spend a large amount of time wondering what life would be like for them if they did not have a disability. To repeat, healthy students are aware of educational choices and accept responsibility for making them.

What about healthy teachers? In addition to displaying traits similar to those of healthy students, healthy teachers are perceptive persons. They do not see everything in dichotomous terms— *good* or *bad, disabled* or *nondisabled, black* or *white,* and so forth. Healthy teachers have insight into the behavior of their students; yet, they do not exploit that insight. They use it to empathize with the needs of students. Such insight gives them the ability to identify vicariously with the successes of students, and with their failures, too.

There seems to be a significant positive correlation between the height of students' self-concept and the degree to which teachers are calm, accepting, supportive, and facilitative. A negative correlation usually is found when teachers are dominating, threatening, and sarcastic. Disabled students who have warm, considerate teachers tend to make sounder decisions, and they are more likely to return for additional education. If teachers have a positive perception of their students, e.g. if they think the students are capable persons, students feel like partners in the learning process.

It is extremely important for teachers and students to be aware of their respective beliefs and value systems. There are four potential problem areas in teachers' beliefs and values pertaining to students:

1. Teachers often are unaware of their beliefs about disabilities until forced to look at them.

2. Some of the teachers' values conflict with those of their friends.

3. The beliefs teachers espouse about people with disabilities are often different from their actions.

4. Some of the teachers' values and beliefs are impossible to realize because they are inconsistent with the facts of students' lives.

Paraphrasing Gilbert Wrenn (1958), the authors offer teachers four suggestions, which are both values and principles to be followed as a basic teaching credo:

1. Strive to see the positive aspects of all students and mention them at least as often that which is to be corrected.

2. If correcting or criticizing students' actions, be sure that this is seen by them as criticism of specific behaviors and not as criticism of themselves as persons.

3. Assume that all students can see some reasonableness in their behavior, that there is meaning in it for them if not for the teacher.

4. When the teacher contributes to students' self-respect, he or she increases their positive feelings toward and their respect for him or her.

SUMMARY

The challenge to teachers is great. They must find a way to overcome their own negative behaviors as well as those of their students. When measured in dollars, the rewards of this task are few, but when measured in professional and personal success, there are many rewards for the more effective teachers. Besides, these teachers try to maximize the education of students with disabilities because it is the right thing to do. The most important lessons all students learn are not those that teachers pontificate but rather the lessons in human relations they give to students simply by behaving as caring people. These are the messages of the self that all caring people send and receive constantly. Self-initiated messages may be conscious or unconscious, direct or indirect, obvious or subtle; they may be conveyed by word, gesture, tone of voice, or look.

NOTE TO HELPERS

Some questions for teachers and other helpers to ask themselves are:

1. Do you help students accept each other on the basis of individual worth, regardless of physical abilities, sex, race, and socioeconomic background? How do you do it?

2. Do you help students to recognize clearly the basic similarities among all members of the human race as well as the uniqueness of every individual? What are some differences and similarities between persons with disabilities and persons without disabilities?

3. Do you help students to value the various physical characteristics of this society and to reject stereotypes or derogatory caricatures of people with disabilities? What do you do?

4. Do you help students to see prejudice as a wall that blocks communication, interaction, mutual understanding, and respect? What intervention would you use if you heard one student call another a cripple?

5. Do you help students to be knowledgeable about pressures—historical and contemporary, environmental, social, political, and economic—that have been instrumental in developing life-styles of people with disabilities? Can you list some of the pressures?

6. Do you help students honestly and objectively to analyze group tension and conflict with a will to resolve destructive situations and to seek fairness, cooperation, and affirmative action? What guidelines do you use?

7. Do you help students to appreciate the contributions of all groups? What are some contributions made by people with disabilities?

8. Do you motivate students to accept their responsibilities as citizens to abate injustices? How do you do this? (If you do not, why don't you?)

9. Do you help students by carefully evaluating before classroom usage all curriculum materials (books, pamphlets, films, filmstrips, bulletin board pictures) to ensure fair and balanced treatment of all groups? Can you name a movie, a book, a film, and a television program that fairly portray persons with disabilities?

10. Do you help students to learn the art of good human relations by providing a living model in your own treatment of people—each and every student, all members of the staff, and other members of the community?

REFERENCES

Allport, Gordon. *The Nature of Prejudice.* Garden City, NJ: Doubleday, 1958.

Banks, George, Berenson, Bernard G., and Carkhuff, Robert R. The effects of counselor race training upon negro clients in initial interviews. *J Clin Psychol, 23:* 70–72, 1967.

Benjamin, Alfred. *The Helping Interview.* Boston: Houghton Mifflin, 1969.

Broadbent, Frank W., and Cruickshank, Donald R. *The Identification and Analysis of Problems of First Year Teachers.* Unpublished paper. State University of New York, 1965.

Buber, Martin. *I and Thou.* New York: Scribners, 1958.

Gordon, Jesse E. *Personality and Behavior.* New York: Macmillan, 1963.

Gordon, Thomas. A theory of healthy relationships and a program of parent effectiveness training. In Hart, J. T., and Tomlinson, T. M. (Eds.). *New Directions in Client-Centered Therapy.* Boston: Houghton Mifflin, 1970.

Hollingshead, August B., and Redlich, Frederick C. *Social Class and Mental Illness.* New York: John Wiley & Sons, 1958.

Jersild, Arthur T. *Education for Understanding.* New York: Columbia University Press, 1953.

Jourard, Sidney M. *Personal Adjustment: An Approach Through the Study of Healthy Personality.* New York: Macmillan, 1963.

Keith-Lucas, Alan. *Giving and Taking Help.* Chapel Hill: University of North Carolina Press, 1972.

Lee, Harper. *To Kill a Mockingbird.* New York: Popular Library, 1960.

Rogers, Carl R. The characteristics of a helping relationship. *Pers Guid J, 37:* 6–14, 1958.

Rogers, Carl R. The process equation of psychotherapy. *Am J Psychother, 15:* 21–45, 1961.

Wrenn, Gilbert C. Psychology, religion, and values for counselors. *Pers Guid J, 36:* 43, 1958.

Additional Readings

Banks, James A. *Teaching Strategies for Ethnic Studies.* Boston: Allyn & Bacon, 1979.

Batshaw, Mark. *Children with Handicaps: A Medical Primer.* Baltimore: Paul H. Brookes, 1981.

Bigge, June L. *Teaching Individuals with Physical and Multiple Disabilities.* Columbus, OH: Charles E. Merrill, 1982.

Brewer, Garry D., and Kakalik, James S. *Handicapped Children: Strategies for Improving Services.* New York: McGraw-Hill, 1979.

Davis, William E. *Educator's Resource Guide to Special Education: Terms — Laws — Organizations.* Rockleigh, NJ: Allyn & Bacon, 1980.

Dixon, Nancy Powell. *Children of Poverty with Handicapping Conditions: How Teachers Can Cope Humanistically.* Springfield, IL: Charles C Thomas, 1981.

Gearheart, William R. *A Teacher's Guide to Management of Physically Handicapped Students.* Springfield, IL: Charles C Thomas, 1979.

Lindsey, Carolyn N., Leibold, Susan R., Ladd, Frances T., and Ownby, Ralph. Children on medications: A guide for teachers. *Rehab Lit, 41:* 124–126, 1980.

Love, Harold D., and Walthall, Joe E. *A Handbook of Medical, Education and Psychological Information for Teachers of Physically Handicapped Children.* Springfield, IL: Charles C Thomas, 1977.

Martin, Reed. *Educating Handicapped Children: The Legal Mandate.* Champaign, IL: Research Press, 1979.

McGuire, William J., McGuire, Clair V., Child, Pamela, and Fryeoka, Terry. Salience of ethnicity in the spontaneous self-concept as a function of one's ethnic distinctiveness in the social environment. *J Pers Soc Psychol, 36:* 511–520, 1978.

Mullins, June B. *A Teacher's Guide to Management of Physically Handicapped Students.* Springfield, IL: Charles C Thomas, 1979.

Ross, Ruth-Ellen K. *Handicapped People in Society: Ideas and Activities for Teachers.* Morristown, NJ: Silver Burdett, 1981.

Smith, William D., Burlew, Ann K., Mosley, Myrtis H., and Whitney, W. Monty. *Minority Issues in Mental Health.* Reading, MA: Addison-Wesley, 1978.

Taylor, Ronald L. Psychosocial development among black children and youth: A re-examination. *Am J Orthopsychiatry, 46:* 4–19, 1976.

Verma, Gajendra, and Bagley, Christopher (Eds.). *Self-Concept, Achievement and Multicultural Education.* London: Macmillan, 1982.

Chapter 10

TIPS FOR OTHER
HUMAN SERVICES PERSONNEL

All people with disabilities are in simultaneous states of *being* and *becoming* something. Whatever they are, they are not stagnant. Even dying is an active process. Those who are being socioeconomic failures would like to become successes, and those who are successful try to be even more successful. A major aspect of the upward quest for adjustment centers on social acceptance by peers. A typical change in status involves shedding the stigma attached to disability. The most obvious status changes are economic ones, whether upward or downward. It is shortsighted to ignore upwardly and downwardly mobile people and focus attention only on individuals and families that are well established in the middle and upper classes.

It is true that there is less social risk working with economically well-established people with disabilities, but it is also true that they are not the largest group. There are more marginal-income than stable-income Americans with disabilities. Moreover, contrary to popular opinion, it is not too late to alter the employment and living conditions of lower-class adults with disabilities. Concerned human services personnel can and do make a difference. This chapter will use adult clients as the treatment group, build on points made in the earlier chapters, and add a few new tips.

PURPOSE OF THE INTERVIEW

Interviews with clients with disabilities serve many purposes, but the major ones are to obtain and give information, to provide clients an opportunity to ventilate their feelings and relieve tension, and to assist clients in understanding and resolving their problems. In order for helpers to be optimally effective, they must have respect for people with disabilities as human beings, not as disabled people. This includes taking into account the clients' needs, problems, fears, and cultural backgrounds. It is important at the outset to give clients credit for having the capacity to select their own solutions or answers. Thus, the job of the helper is not to solve clients' problems but instead to strengthen their ability to do so.

The success of any interview depends primarily on the helper's ability to establish and maintain a healthy interpersonal relationship with the client. The attainment of such a relationship is to a great extent based on intangibles such as warmth, sensitivity, and interest. Speech alone is seldom adequate to convey these traits. To all but the visually impaired client, the helper's physical appearance, movement, facial expressions, and demeanor—all convey acceptance or rejection. Touch is also an important aspect of the helping relationship.

The major task of human services personnel is to help clients adjust to their problems. This means guiding them to information pertaining to their disabilities and attitudes about themselves and other people. Effectively listening as the client speaks is one of the most valuable tools available to a helper. What at first glance appears to be a natural process is in fact a deceptively difficult art that must be learned. It seems easy, but effective listening requires helpers to put aside their own personal needs to talk, explore things, and solve personal problems in order to assist someone else. Most conversations are barely listened to. For most people, hearing is natural, but listening is not. Attending to the verbal and nonverbal communications of clients with disabilities is an art and a skill that most helpers learn on the job, if they learn it at all. The sensitive helper knows that clients with physical disabilities need more than physical rehabilitation. A successful interview can provide the client with a rare opportunity to be heard in a noncritical setting.

A DELICATE BALANCE

Physical disability is a social, mental, and physiological condition. Much of the job of the helper is to assist or accompany clients as they deal with discrimination, rejection, and low social status. Sometimes these problems are overt, but most often they are covert. Specific goals of helping include:

1. Reaffirming to clients the fact that they are people first and people with disabilities second

2. Assisting clients to understand the physiological facts and social issues involved in their disabling conditions

3. Encouraging clients to deal with their feelings centering on being disabled

4. Aiding clients to accept their disabilities emotionally and intellectually without devaluing themselves

Clients with disabilities are people, not things to be manipulated. Sometimes they are fragile people—frightened, confused, and defensive—but they are seldom "sick" people. Helpers should not be impatient or insensitive to their hurts, fears, and hostility. Chapter 9 talked about empathy, congruence, and unconditional positive regard. These concepts apply here, too. Like teachers, other helpers should be guides, not gods. The more effective helpers acknowledge their own humanity, but too often, professional helpers forget that people with disabilities are, as Karl Menninger (1942) pointed out, people: "The world is made up of people, but the people of the world forget this. It is hard to believe that, like ourselves, other people are born of women, reared by parents, teased by brothers, . . . consoled by wives, . . . flattered by grandchildren, and buried by parsons and priests with the blessings of the church and the tears of those left behind" (p. 114).

The words inscribed on a plaque hanging in the office of a professional helper are also instructive: "I feel so much better, less helpless and guilty, since I found out I was not chosen to be God." All humans fail from time to time. This is not the worst that can happen to helpers or their clients, if they admit their failures and, where appropriate, refer clients they cannot help to someone they think can. Throughout the helping process, neither the identity of the helper nor that of the client with a disability must be destroyed.

> To incorporate another person is to swallow him up, to overwhelm him; and thus to treat him ultimately as less than a whole person. To identify with another person is to lose oneself, to submerge one's own identity in that of the other, to be overwhelmed, and hence to treat oneself ultimately as less than a whole person. To pass judgment . . . is to place oneself in an attitude of superiority; to agree offhandandly is to place oneself in an attitude of inferiority. . . . The personality can cease to exist in two ways— either by destroying the other, or being absorbed by the other—and maturity in interpersonal relationships demands that neither oneself nor the other shall disappear, but that each shall contribute to the affirmation and realization of the other's personality. [Storr, 1961, pp. 41–43]

It is of crucial importance that those involved in the helping relationship avoid labeling, stereotyping, and rationalizing away the unique person who defies reduction and simplification. Behavioral sciences theories certainly have their place and have provided invaluable heuristic tools for helpers to use. Even so, helpers must be willing to discard these theoretical devices when they do not fit the situation or when they cease to provide understanding of individuals or groups of persons with disabilities. M. Esther Harding (1965) is correct: "We cannot change anyone else; we can change only ourselves, and then usually only when the elements that are in need of reform have become conscious through their reflection in someone else" (p. 75).

Helpers must be in touch with and have grasp of what is going on within their own selves before they can help their clients to make choices. Whether they are involved in a helping relationship as professionals, paraprofessionals, or friends and confidantes, it is inevitable that at some point in the relationship the problem of making choices will arise. Helping relationships in which choosing is being continually delayed or postponed by the helper and avoided or procrastinated by the client should be seriously questioned. All too often the helper is meeting his or her own needs by being too protective and not allowing the client to experience the pain and discomfort that generally accompany choosing between alternatives.

Søren Kierkegaard (1962), the father of contemporary existentialist philosophy, described the task of the helping person in this manner: "The highest one human being can do for another is to make the other free, to help him to stand on his own feet — alone. . . . When a person has overcome all, precisely then is he perhaps closest to losing everything . . . no longer can he fight against something or someone else . . . now he must stand alone" (p. 22).

In summary, there is a delicate balance between helping and doing. Clients with disabilities must be allowed to do all that they can for themselves with the assistance of the helper. The work of the professional includes helping them to fill a need, receive a service, and otherwise solve or resolve a problem. The core material of the helping relationship is interaction of the basic attitudes and emotions of the helper and client. All clients need the following: to be treated as individuals, to be allowed to express their feelings, to receive empathic responses, to be allowed to make choices and decisions, and to have their secrets kept.

In order to help their clients, human services personnel must be willing to learn from them, to discover not only their weaknesses but also their strengths. First, helpers must learn what a client knows and would like to know, and what he or she can do, cannot do, and would like to do. Second, helpers must be astute observers of role behaviors. This means analyzing the actions and reactions between people; sorting out their attitudes, values, and beliefs; and understanding the emotions underlying human behavior. Roles are never static, not even the role of "cripple."

PEOPLE WHO CARE

The various styles of helping that professionals and para-professionals use when interacting with clients have been described in many ways, including *authoritarian, democratic* and *laissez-faire.* Authoritarian helpers unilaterally set goals for their clients. Furthermore, they collect all the information and make all the arrangements without permitting their clients to assist in planning. Authoritarian helpers produce a great deal of work-oriented behavior but a low degree of personal involvement. Furthermore, clients who have authoritarian helpers tend to be easily discouraged.

Democratic helpers attempt to identify their clients' goals and needs and allow them to assist actively in the initial planning as well as subsequent action. As would be expected, client morale is high with democratic helpers. Laissez-faire helpers assume no active participation and allow clients to do whatever they want; most or all of the initiative is left to the clients. As might be expected, the laissez-faire helper is the least effective of the three.

Effective helpers assist clients to succeed in achieving their goals while at the same time minimizing their failures. The *authority role* of the helper need not be synonymous with *domination*. Some clients are not cooperative merely because they do not like authority in any form. Needless to say, helpers determined to "show these people who's boss" are likely to discover obstinate and recalcitrant individuals who would rather fail than be treated in this manner. For this reason, a helper's behavior should say to the client, "I am here to understand you so that I can help you." This type of authority extends beyond finding fault and prescribing cures. Clients with disabilities need to feel that their helpers understand and accept them as unique individuals with value beyond a promotion or a day's work. In the end, the respect clients have for a helper will be determined by how successful the helper is in assisting them to adjust to their unique situations.

Individuals who do not feel accepted and wanted will find it extremely difficult to relate to helpers in a positive manner. They may withdraw, not pay attention in conferences, complain easily, not provide needed information, miss appointments and, finally, terminate the relationship. When this happens, clients appear to have no interest in completing the helping process. In reality, they have little or no interest in completing the process *with their current helpers.* Their uncooperative behavior is a not-too-subtle way of breaking off a relationship so that they can try to find more suitable helpers. Thus, it should be evident that rejection works two ways. Not only do human services personnel reject people with disabilities, but people with disabilities reject insensitive would-be helpers, too.

Successful helpers are able to give of themselves and unconditionally receive their clients. The act of unconditional acceptance communicates to the disabled: "I acknowledge your physical differences. I am here to help meet your needs, but I will not cause you to lose your self-esteem." Acceptance does not, however, mean feeling *like* individuals with disabilities or anyone else, but it does mean feeling *with* them. No individual can feel like another because no two persons live in the same cognitive world. However, by trying, human services personnel can understand the environmental forces having impact on the lives of persons with disabilities. The best way to get a feeling for clients' living conditions is to visit their homes, walk around their neighborhoods, visit their friends, talk with neighborhood merchants, and read current books and journals focusing on disabilities.

An optimum helper-helpee relationship involves two people freely responding to each other. This does not mean that the relationship will always be pleasant or comfortable. Rather, it is a relationship in which both parties feel free to say, "I agree" or "I disagree." There are two important ways this open, honest interaction can be beneficial to persons with disabilities who live as second-class citizens in their respective communities. First, helpers can assist them to differentiate between opportunities available in their neighborhoods and those available in the larger community. Second, helpers can assist disabled individuals to acquire needed skills and resources. This, then, is an action-oriented approach to helping. To be successful, it requires open, honest communication.

Channels of communication are open only when helpers uncritically accept each client's efforts to communicate. This means learning to "hear" nonverbal communication such as sighs, frowns, and smiles. Obviously this kind of understanding comes from being familiar with each client's background and disability. While the negative effects of a person's physical or environmental restrictions cannot be completely erased, they can be ameliorated by offering hope in the place of despair and confidence instead of insecurity. It is important to remember that most people with disabilities are very sensitive to what helpers do *not* say as well as what they do say. The key is not to give up on persons before trying to understand and help them.

Nonverbal communication should never be considered an acceptable substitute for words unless the client is deaf. Nonverbal communication is commonly called *body language*. Technically, it is the science of *kinesics.* This science includes the study of reflexive and nonreflexive movements of a part or all of the body used by a person to communicate a message. There are several kinds of body language that helpers use, including the following:

GESTURES AND CLUSTERS OF GESTURES. There are approximately 1 million distinct gestures that have meaning to people around the world. They are produced by facial expressions, postures, and movements of the arms, hands, legs, and so forth. Gestures are essential face-to-face communication.

MANNER OF SPEAKING. The tone of a helper's voice, the placing of oral emphasis, is closely related to gestures. Specifically, the manner of speaking includes the quality, volume, pitch, and duration of speech. Indeed, how a message is delivered greatly influences clients.

ZONES OF TERRITORY. Edward Hall (1959) coined the term *proxemics* to describe human zones of spatial territory and how they are used. Zones of movement increase as intimacy decreases. That is, the more space available without other persons present, the more movement is likely to occur. In informal gatherings, a distance of six to eighteen inches is considered too close for the average white American male without a disability, whereas this distance does not cause discomfort for the average person with a disability or for white females without disabilities.

EYE CONTACT. Most Americans are taught not to stare at other people. Instead, they learn to acknowledge another person's presence through deliberate and polite inattention. That is, they look long enough to make it clear that they see the other person and then look away. Most professional helpers are taught to stare at clients—even if it embarrasses them.

TOUCHING. The sense of touch conveys acceptance or rejection, warmth or coldness, positive or negative feelings. This is the single most difficult aspect of nonverbal communication for helpers dealing with clients who have disabilities. Most helpers devise ingenious ways to occupy their hands so as to avoid touching persons with physical disabilities.

LISTENING. Effective helping does not occur unless effective listening also occurs. Agency interviews are designed to get and give information. It is during the interview that listening skills become crucial to diagnosis.

Caring about clients is based on the premise that the primary emphasis within the helping process should be on cooperation rather than control. Helpers who become preoccupied with filling out forms, improving their pep talks, and maintaining rigid time schedules are not likely to be flexible enough to help people with disabilities. Successful helpers are able to provide both *structure* and *freedom* during the helping process. In short, they are able to stay loose and still provide adequate guidance. It is one thing to know what someone needs to do; it is something else to devise a way to help him or her to do it.

The helper who understands people is better able to win their confidence and perceive alternatives for meeting their needs. This kind of helper does not join the local Quitter's Club, whose members look forward to and devise unhelpful methods for terminating relationships with physically impaired persons. The major goal of quitters is to get these clients into the first activity or situation available, even if it is not what they want or need. Caring primarily about their own discomfort, these helpers are basically negative about interacting with people with disabilities, whom they believe to be ugly and of low status. Individuals who are obsessed with sorting out physical abilities, colors, races, and social classes are not likely to treat all people fairly. They cannot assure rejected clients that they care about them, because they do not. Helpers who really care about people are not uncomfortable around individuals because of their physical conditions, color, or ethnic identity.

Since most people enter the helping relationship wanting to be accepted, to be accepted by human services personnel is a sign of their social worth, and to be accepted by a helper they like and respect causes them to feel very special. Clients who feel the need to move away from helpers are frightened, and those who believe they must move against them are angry. Both types of behavior are easily triggered by human services personnel who do not care. There are obvious risks in caring about clients, however. The temporary nature of most helper-helpee relationships is stressful for both parties. This is compounded by the fact that some persons have physical and psychological limitations that no helper can alter. To care under these conditions is to become frustrated by an inability to succeed.

Some minority-group helpers are afraid to care about persons with disabilities because they believe they will lose their newly achieved middle-class status. For example, some black Americans with disabilities are unwilling to work with lower-class blacks with disabilities. These black Anglo-Saxons do not want to be identified with poor people, especially poor black people with disabilities. Their self-hatred becomes intensified when community norms force them to live in neighborhoods with lower-class black people. Minority-group helpers who reject their own ethnic identity are not likely to be cultural bridges between themselves and other people.

ESTABLISHING RAPPORT

Anger about their perceived low status causes some persons with disabilities to view every professional worker who does not have a disability with deep suspicion, i.e. the hearing-impaired are constantly on their guard around professionals who are not hearing impaired. In addition, the rise in consciousness of minority-group people involved in civil rights activities initially heightens their feelings of distrust of the nonmembers. Extreme cases of distrust result in the erroneous belief that only helpers with the same disability as the clients' are qualified to work with them, e.g. helpers with visual impairments with clients who have visual impairments, hearing-impaired helpers with hearing-impaired people, and so forth. Such an elitist, exclusionary view is not one that the authors of this book support.

The challenge to the human services worker is to demonstrate that competence and empathy are not traits unique to persons with a particular disability. For example, a competent helper can, when judged by his or her deeds, be a kindred soul to all clients. A disability is more than a physical condition. It is thinking, behaving, and accepting the disability. When this happens, people with disabilities admit that some helpers without disabilities have "soul." Relatedly, competent helpers with disabilities have been able to prove to clients who do not have disabilities that they have soul, too. Physical disability is neither a guarantee of nor an automatic deterrent to establishing rapport with clients. Attitudes and human relations skills are more important factors.

The first step in establishing rapport with clients is to help them relax. In order to do this, the helper must be relaxed. When helpers do not know how to communicate with clients, neither party will relax. Instead, helpers will hide behind their desks and academic degrees, and clients will hide behind their disabilities. Both helpers and clients who behave this way believe the media stereotypes of persons with disabilities being inferior or strange people. Thus, the discomfort of helpers can produce feelings of discomfort in their clients. During these stressful periods, conversation related to educational or technical subjects may panic the clients. Yet, it is precisely these subjects that the helper is likely to feel most comfortable discussing. A few minutes of informal talk can often reduce the stress. A warm, informal, down-to-earth approach to each person is a prerequisite to establishing rapport. The message to helpers is: "Don't fake it. Be yourself — that is, be your warm, caring self, if you have one."

Some clients approach professional helpers in ways that are outright defensive. Those using defensive mechanisms usually do not have faulty personalities. Instead, it is their environment that is faulty. Protection of the ego is normal, but a disproportionate use of defenses indicates a lack of security. Clients with disabilities who imagine that they are objects of rejection or ridicule develop rigid, persistent, and chronic ego-protection devices. Continued feelings of rejection result in behavior inappropriate to reality. This behavior was demonstrated by a client who imagined that his rehabilitation counselor disliked him. To protect himself, he withdrew from all voluntary contact with her. One day the counselor asked him, "Why do you avoid me?" The client answered, "Because you don't like me. You smile at the nondisabled people and joke with them, but you never do these things with me."

Issues that center on disabilities cause many helpers to overreact. Often it is difficult to sift out fact from fiction, objectivity from subjectivity, but it must be done. The development of excessive ego defenses by the client is disturbing to helpers who are unaware of having done anything to elicit such behavior. A smile or an approving nod are small but often effective ways to communicate acceptance and break down the defensive barriers. Asking individuals what is bothering them provides them with an opportunity to get some things out in the open. The key is to try to establish rapport. Sometimes clients need love and acceptance most when they are most unloving and unaccepting of others.

The willingness of clients to continue interacting with professionals and paraprofessionals who want to help them is affected in part by the attractiveness of the arrangement (What is in it for them?) and in part by the belief that only through a cooperative effort can they achieve certain goals. In short, there must be some real or imagined payoff when they cooperate with helpers. The old "do as I tell you because I am the expert" approach works only if clients are intimidated by the helper's status. Open, honest expressions of feelings obviate the necessity for hidden anger. Indeed, freedom of expression should be not only allowed but encouraged.

An *open dialogue* is not synonymous with *automatic approval*, however. Helpers should make it clear that encouraging candid expressions of feelings does not mean that they necessarily agree with the feelings verbalized. Such conversations or dialogues will probably be a new experience for many persons with physical disabilities. People without disabilities seldom ask people with disabilities what they think; they usually tell them what they should be thinking. Thus, when asked to participate in uncritical discussions, many clients with disabilities will be unprepared and even hesitant. However, once they start talking, the danger is not that they will be silent again but that they may not stop talking. Good helpers are good listeners. They learn to listen with all their senses, not merely their ears.

The first concerns expressed by clients may not be the ones they really want to discuss. That is, they may want to talk about sex or school or a job rather than physical disabilities *per se.* In the end, whatever pressing problems a person brings to a helper are the ones he or she will discuss, one way or another. It is not enough to encourage an open discussion; helpers must also accept the client's views. The attention of a reticent client has been compared to a wild animal that must be lured, caught, and held. Along with honest dialogue, the helper must show interest and involvement. Nods and blank stares from the helper are not always interpreted by clients as understanding. It is important for the helper to communicate what he or she understands and what the client needs to do.

People with disabilities cannot respond with conforming behavior if they do not know what is expected of them. Helpers should not be like the near-hysterical beginning teacher who rushed into the principal's office and cried, "This is the last straw. I quit. Those kids are sleeping and running all over the room. I can't control them." The principal thought for a minute, then asked, "Have you told them to sit up, sit down, and be quiet?" As if struck by a bolt of insight, the teacher ran out of the office and back to the classroom. She had been so eager to begin the lesson that she had forgotten to call the class to order. Similar to students in a class, some clients are apathetic, low in energy output, and passive in behavior. Others are impulsive, hyperactive, and diffuse in behavior. It is this wide range of behaviors that makes it impossible to characterize people with disabilities and illustrates why helpers should refrain from stereotyping them.

BEYOND TELLING

When a permanent disability is diagnosed, many individuals grieve. Helpers should be aware of their stages of grief, which are similar to those of terminally ill patients:

1. *Denial and isolation* — refusal to accept the permanence of their disabilities and desire to be alone

2. *Anger* at professionals and friends for giving up on them

3. *Bargaining* — trying to strike a deal with God or some other supernatural force by stating that they will do something good in exchange for restoration of the body function or limbs

4. *Depression* — a sense of loss and realization that they are permanently disabled and, finally, for most persons,

5. *Acceptance* of their disabilities.

It is important to know what stage the client is in.

During the early stages of grieving, a clients' attitudes and behavior may change from day to day: Yesterday they wanted to talk about their disability; today they deny that they are disabled. It is therapeutic for helpers to elicit emotional expression rather than emotional repression. A free exchange of thoughts is the beginning of the rehabilitation process. It is of utmost importance to know what the client is feeling. Physicians usually can relieve the physiological symptoms of a disability, but other helpers are needed to relieve the psychological pain from the loss of body image and self-esteem. Family members and friends can help in this process. Effective helping occurs within the context of environment, culture, social roles, and power.

ENVIRONMENT. It is necessary only to look around in order to see how the physical environment affects the quality of the helper-helpee interaction, considering the differences between inner-city slums and affluent suburbs, mountains and seashores, chemically polluted and nonpolluted communities. Environments are equivalent to nonverbal statements about health care: They cause clients and their helpers to feel fearful or relaxed, cheerful or sad, open or closed.

CULTURE. Culture preference is a major problem in most helper-helpee interactions. Members of different cultures live in different worlds. Inability to understand and communicate with culturally different persons renders would-be helpers therapeutically impotent. It is culture more than disability that stands between helpers and clients.

SOCIAL ROLES. Shakespeare said it well in *As You Like It:* "All the world's a stage./And all men and women merely players./They have their exits and their entrances, And one man in his time plays many parts." Some helpers forget that "professional" is a role and not themselves. Conversely, "handicapped" is a role and not the essence of the individual so labeled. Inflexible role players are unable to change when solutions require role adaptation.

POWER. It is clear that most helpers have a degree of power over clients. As noted earlier, helpers who are authoritarian and dominating tend to be less helpful than their colleagues who are democratic and encourage client initiative. Part of the helpers' dilemma is that they must be sufficiently detached from clients to exercise sound judgment and at the same time have enough concern to provide sensitive, empathic care. It is possible for professional helpers to suppress on a conscious level emotional responses while counseling and assisting clients, but this detachment does not remove the stress and concern hidden in the unconscious domain of their minds. The pathological process of detachment that tends to produce mature helpers also tends to produce cynical clinicians.

Helping clients with disabilities to tell what they feel requires more than a receptive listener, and it is more than collecting predetermined data. Helpers who believe that the predetermined interview schedule is the only effective method of eliciting pertinent data should learn from the experiences of social workers. Helen Perlman (1957) wrote:

> It has long been said in casework, reiterated against the sometime practice of subjecting the client to a barrage of ready-made questions, that the client "should be allowed to tell his story in his own way." Particularly at the beginning this is true, because the client may feel an urgency to do just that, to pour out what *he* sees and thinks and feels because it is his problem and because he has lived with it and mulled it within himself for days or perhaps months. Moreover, it is "his own way" that gives both caseworker and client not just the objective facts of the problem, but the grasp of its significance. To the client who is ready and able to "give out" with what troubles him, the caseworker's nods and murmurs of understanding—any of those nonverbal ways by which we indicate response—may be all the client needs in his first experience of telling and being heard out. [P. 142]

Not all clients can easily talk about their disabilities. Comments such as "I imagine that this is not easy for you to talk about" and "Go on, I'm listening" may be enough encouragement for some reticent persons. Others will need direct questions to help them focus their conversation. Accurate information is not the result of passive listening; it is the by-product of interpretive talking and active listening. Effective listening is demanding; most people have to work hard at listening to hear what others are trying to say.

Few people know exactly how they feel about their disabilities until they have communicated sufficient data to another person. To tell someone what and how they feel is in itself a relief for many clients, but telling is not enough. Problem resolution must follow if the helping relationship is to be complete. This is likely to occur when the client's questions pertaining to his or her problem are amply discussed. The words of Paul Tournier (1957) sum up the process of helping persons with disabilities to communicate: "Through information I can understand a case, only through communication shall I be able to understand a person" (p. 25).

The dynamics of problem solving are threefold. First, the facts that surround the disability must be understood. Facts frequently consist of objective reality and subjective reactions to it. Second, the facts must be thought through. They must be probed into, reorganized, and turned over in order for the client to grasp as much of the total configuration as possible. Third, a plan must be devised that will result in some type of adjustment.

Fact finding is more complex than many authors suggest. Seldom are professional helpers taught to elicit information—how to talk, to listen, and to provide feedback. However, this does not mean that there are only a few professionals who can communicate effectively with people with disabilities. There are many who do so, but most of them are self-taught. Something as important as communication should not be left to intuition or chance. It should be a part of all college curricula and in-service training programs.

Numerous studies have concluded that a large number of persons with disabilities receive insufficient information about their conditions and coping skills. For example, many persons terminate agency relationships without ever having understood what their helpers decided were their needs, why certain procedures were followed, what, if anything, their failures consisted of, and what the reasons for them were. The rights of clients include the right to courteous, prompt, and the best treatment. They also include the right to know what is wrong, why, and what can be done about it. A case could be built that this ignorance is a by-product of the helping mystique. That is, professional and lay helpers typically are perceived as being men and women whose training and predilections place them in a special service category. To put it even more bluntly, there is a tendency for clients to be in awe of individuals who help them. This intangible dimension of the helping process is one reason, but attention must be given to other reasons communication breaks down.

There are many reasons for an individual's failure to communicate pertinent information. Some persons with disabilities make no effort to communicate information about their situation. In other instances, helpers fail to request needed information, particularly that which would give them basic understanding of the individual with a disability. Since human communication is a two-way process, both helpers and clients distort messages. Some individuals forget information that had been clearly communicated to them.

Furthermore, research demonstrating that people who understand their illness adjust more quickly than those who do not is sparse. From this narrow perspective one could conclude that clients' understanding of their disabilities is unimportant. However, if a goal of helping is educating or informing people, then it is important for clients to understand what is happening to them. In the end, the quality of the information helpers are able to give is directly proportional to the quality of information they solicit. Additional tips for facilitating the communication process are as follows:

1. Respect the family. In most instances, the family is very much involved in decisions made by disabled members. The final decision may be made by the client, but only after considering the feelings of other family members.
2. Call people by their right names. In Spanish, for example, each person has two last names. The first last name is the father's family name, and the second last name is the mother's family name. Use both last names so as not to insult the client. Also, use the correct pronunciation of names.
3. Try to understand local customs.
4. Analyze your feelings about various physical disabilities.
5. Avoid patronizing or condescending approaches.
6. When giving information, do not merely ask if clients understand what you have said. Ask them to tell you what they think you have said.

In the end, the most successful helpers are linguistically compatible with their clients, empathic, and well trained. This means that the initial edge held by a helper with the same disability or from the same ethnic group as the client will be lost if he or she cannot go beyond physical identity and ethnicity. A helper does not have to have a disability in order to assist people with disabilities effectively.

CONFERENCE ETIQUETTE

Human services workers should not jump to false conclusions when some clients arrive late to their appointments. It is possible that because of their disabilities they have seldom been asked to be on time by their parents or friends. Thus, the term *C.P. (crippled people) time* connotes being chronically late. Interestingly, there are many people without disabilities who are chronically late to meetings, too. This does not mean that they cannot be punctual if asked to be. When clients do arrive on time, human services workers should not show surprise by commending them for being punctual, and certainly they should not be like the teacher who began a school program by announcing, "This is truly an historic occasion. You parents have proven that Indians can be on time."

Agency personnel also should not be surprised if individuals with physical disabilities do not exhibit psychopathic or sociopathic personalities. Most people with disabilities are quite normal. Many of them have adapted to the realities of their limited physical abilities and restricted social and employment opportunities.

The first impressions a client forms of a helper are frequently lasting impressions. During the first meeting, the professional helper should welcome clients, shake their hands, call them by their names, and introduce himself or herself. Whether or not to shake hands with females (if they have hands) is not so much an issue as is the type of handshake. A limp, spongy handshake is hardly the way to communicate acceptance to males or females. Helpers must treat all clients with respect and speak to them with words they can understand. Talking over someone's head or in a patronizing manner, i.e. "Honey, you'll like this" or "Sweetie, the depreciation of this property can be enough to capitalize a bond investment," is not an effective way to build rapport. The more effective helpers keep the conversation simple and to the point, and they get technical only when necessary or the client asks technical questions.

Each conference should begin with a topic that is pleasant.

However, caution should be taken not to delay too long before beginning to discuss the matter at hand. In any case, the helper should begin the discussion by focusing on the client's assets. In addition to being reassuring, this approach is likely to evoke minimum stress and less defensiveness. In order to be successful, helpers should clearly delineate information that is needed and steps to be followed in trying to achieve rehabilitation goals. Communication based on concrete problems or issues generally is productive, while conversation that is abstract and vague tends to be anxiety producing. Once rapport is established, the client may volunteer personal and embarrassing data. This information must be kept in the utmost confidence.

When helpers visit clients' homes, they should arrange for the visit well in advance. Most people tend to resent individuals' "popping in" just to be friendly. Unannounced visits may disrupt the household routine as well as embarrass or anger people. While not an absolute necessity, it is helpful if helpers who visit homes in which English is the second language are able to speak the client's first language, e.g. Spanish. Also, before making home visits, helpers should learn the social codes of the community. This will prevent gossip and needless errors in judgment. In some communities it is taboo for males to visit a married couple's home if the husband is absent. In other communities it is considered bad manners to refuse to drink or eat food that is offered, no matter how unattractive the refreshments may look. The helper who refuses to sit down or play with young children is frowned upon in most communities. Visiting clients requires adhering to their norms. Emerson was correct in saying that "good manners are made up of petty sacrifices."

There are many valid reasons helpers may visit clients' homes, including (1) to inquire about their health, (2) to obtain additional information needed to complete the analysis, (3) to see what their current needs consist of, and (4) to tell them about new opportunities for economic or physical improvement. It is essential that family members and helpers know the purpose of the visit. In all instances, helpers should behave as guests. This does not mean being solicitous, but it does mean being polite.

OPTIMALLY EFFECTIVE HELPERS

Optimally effective helpers are able to manage their negative feelings. This is to imply not that they are completely objective and treat all clients as equals but that they minimize unfair treatment and maximize fair treatment. Getting to know persons with disabilities may not alter negative attitudes toward them but it will enable one to respond better to them. While it would be ideal, a helper need not like persons with disabilities in order to be of assistance to them. Understanding and empathy can occur without condoning or liking.

There are no truly homogeneous groups of persons with disabilities. As seen in Chapter 5, within each ethnic group there are rich and poor, cooperative and uncooperative, dependent and independent. Poverty or affluence *per se* are not absolute determinants of cultural disadvantages or advantages. It is true that poverty-stricken people with disabilities are usually denied adequate socioeconomic opportunities. It is also true that some affluent people do not take advantage of available opportunities. Differences in physical abilities, race, color, or national origin do not in themselves result in a particular condition. For example, black Americans are not as a group subjected to the same kinds of socialization as middle-class white Anglo-Saxon Protestants (WASPs), but neither are other groups. Puerto Ricans, Mexican Americans, American Indians, Asian Americans, and poor whites who do not speak "correct" English are also disadvantaged when competing with WASPs. However, cultural *difference* should not be equated with cultural *deprivation*. None of these groups are deprived of culture.

The quality of human relations within the helper-helpee relationship can be measured by many variables, including how well helpers get along with each other and their clients. One of the first prerequisites for a smoothly functioning helping situation is that persons with disabilities feel welcome and accepted. Without a doubt, the helper is the key person in establishing this atmosphere. People with disabilities should be given the same courteous treatment as all other people. Usually, it is their bodies that are impaired, not their minds or sense of equity. Helpers can find almost anything they want in their clients: Mr. Smith, the loudmouth, is merely the other side of Mr. Smith, the insecure person. When looking at a client, some helpers see only dirty or clean clothes, neat or unkempt hair, straight or twisted bodies. They do not see people. Even worse, they do not accept clients for what they are: people in need of the best help available. Rejection of this kind causes clients to feel like inferior beings who somehow must emerge as "normal" people. Only a body transplant can bring about this feat!

Clients with disabilities in a therapeutically helpful agency environment see themselves as important. What magic will allow helpers to cause this to happen?—None! It does not require magic, only common sense, human relations skills, and patience. These are the hallmark characteristics of optimally effective helpers. They are able to accept disabled people as they are. They are not shocked by what they see or what their clients say. Relatedly, they are able to reject inappropriate *behavior* but not the *persons.* Dual standards are not used, and all clients know what is expected of them. Because they know that identical behavior can come from diverse causes, optimally effective helpers avoid making snap judgments. In short, their ethics are situational.

There are many ways clients may respond in crises situations. Some withdraw, shutting out the world around them; for them the only reality is their imagination, the world within themselves. They may think about the "good old days" when they were younger and there seemed to be fewer problems associated with their disabilities. Others ignore the crisis, refusing to acknowledge that they have problems. Some clients even believe that the only problems people with disabilities have are in the minds of other persons who are trying to stir up trouble (the radicals). The majority of clients with disabilities seek constructive solutions to their problems. They are not immobilized by self-pity, despair, euphoria, or anger.

The human relations problems confronting professional helpers and paraprofessionals are varied and awesome. A quick summary of the seemingly insurmountable and rapidly worsening problems that persons with disabilities face can all but immobilize the best-meaning helpers. Yet, even though they have been shocked awake by the world's imperfections, effective helpers know that standing wide-eyed in horror is an inadequate stance to assume. If human services personnel and their clients are to find solutions, they must forsake the posture of untrained, traumatized innocents. The options are clear: They can either hire out as mourners or try to become actively involved in abating and preventing social problems associated with physical disabilities. Professional and lay helpers must become the realists about whom Malcom Boyd (1971) wrote:

> Shallow activism must . . . be changed into a considerably deeper and more sophisticated sense of involvement. This calls for listening to people outside one's own ingrown and myopic clique as well as sober examination of self-righteousness in one's motives and actions. . . . A realist throws away rose-colored glasses, straightens his shoulder and looks freely about him in all directions. He wants to see whatever there is to see, in relation to other people and things as well as to himself. A realist alone comprehends hope. Optimism is as antithetical to authentic hope as pessimism. Hope is rooted in realism. [P. 128]

Commitment to social change means not *dis*order but a *new* order. Human services personnel do not remain detached, objective, and neutral—far from it—for they are first of all human beings, with their own sets of values, attitudes, beliefs, fears, and dreams, not supermen and superwomen. They are individuals who are superperceptive and untiring in their efforts to eradicate discriminatory behaviors. They do not do this because it will get them a letter of commendation or a promotion. They do it because it is morally, socially, and legally right. They could no more cease trying to bridge cultural gaps than cease being themselves.

There is a bit of skeptic in the more effective helpers. They do not believe that time will take care of things or that most people would not be prejudiced against people with disabilities if they lived with them. Time, they know, is a neutral concept and takes care of nothing. People take care of things. They also know that human services workers do not have to be college trained in order to understand and help people with disabilities. They merely need to care about them and seek out relevant information and experiences. There seems to be some intangible feature that separates effective helpers from ineffective ones. Words such as *under-standing, acceptance,* and *caring* do not adequately describe the inner stuff of this characteristic. One thing seems certain: Optimally effective helpers are not gods and goddesses; they are human beings who somehow manage to climb above the inhumanity surrounding them and help their disabled neighbors to do the same.

FINALLY, SELF-ACTUALIZATION

The only way to help ourselves is by helping others, for as Martin Buber (1957) surmised: "He who calls forth the helping word in himself experiences the world. He who offers support strengthens the support to himself. He who effects salvation to him salvation is disclosed" (p. 110). From this perspective, there is a Godlike quality in helping other people, especially people with disabilities. Buber defined *God* as one who gives meaning to personal life, the being who makes persons capable of meeting, associating with, and helping one another. It is clear that, whether or not they acknowledge it, some agency personnel behave like malevolent gods when determining who shall not be helped. By assisting disabled clients to get an adequate education, housing, jobs, and self-esteem, helpers help themselves and other persons to self-actualize.

Abraham Maslow (1970) described what he called a *hierarchy of needs* peculiar to human beings. The most basic needs are the physiological ones that sustain the body, such as food and sleep. When they are satisfied, the human organism begins to concentrate on fulfilling a need for safety, which usually is accomplished best in an environment that is structured in an orderly and secure fashion. Not until the basic physiological and safety needs are satisfied do people turn their attention to fulfilling their needs for affection, love, and belonging. For helpers to self-actualize, they must do what only they as unique persons can do to help other people. What are the characteristics of these rare people? How can they be recognized? What kind of behavior do they manifest? Maslow (1971) gave an almost poetic description of them:

Self-actualizing people are, without one single exception, involved in a cause outside their skin, in something which fate has called them to somehow and which they work at and which they love, so that the work-joy dichotomy in them disappears. One devoted his life to the laws, another to justice, another to beauty or truth. All, in one way or another, devote their lives to what I have called the "being values" ("B" for short), the ultimate values which are intrinsic, which cannot be reduced to anything more ultimate. There are about fourteen of these B-values, including truth and beauty, and goodness of the ancients and perfection, simplicity, comprehensiveness, and several more. [P. 43]

SUMMARY

In order to help clients achieve their goals, optimally effective helpers are first able to take care of themselves. The people being helped can comprehend the "wholeness" or "togetherness" in these persons. Each success for a client is a personal success for the helper. In the words of Robert Carkhuff (1969): "In a real sense then, the helping process is a process of personal emergence and/or re-emergence. It is a process in which each barrier looms higher than the last, but one in which the rewarding experiences of surmounting previous hurdles increases the probability of future successes. If the helper is not committed to his own physical, emotional, and intellectual development, he cannot enable another to find fulfillment in any or all of these realms of functioning" (p. 31). The authors of this book do not agree with Carkhuff's last assertion. Human services personnel can effectively help clients without taking care of their own needs. However, the price is quite high: Burnout usually occurs. While no one wishes burnout for everyone, there is something ennobling about burning out while trying to help other people.

NOTE TO HELPERS

Problem solving consists of three operations: fact-finding, analysis of facts, and implementation of action steps. To achieve greater effectiveness, persons with disabilities must be fully involved in efforts to solve their problems. It is possible for professionals to define the problems and prescribe the solutions, but this weakens their clients' self-responsibility. After all, clients own the problems; their helpers do not. The following principles are crucial to problem solving:

1. *A problem can be solved only if the necessary resources are available.* A helper may want to understand people with disabilities but be unable to do so because he or she does not have adequate resources, e.g. reading materials. Most helpers are unable to learn about people with disabilities because of missing or inadequate resources. In any puzzle, if pieces are missing, one cannot see the whole picture.

2. *Many clients do not know how they feel about their disability until they communicate their feelings to someone.* They may be vaguely aware of internal discomforts but totally unaware of their implications. Providing clients an opportunity to tell how they feel is usually the first step to isolating negative feelings. Some clients will communicate internal discomforts in a childlike manner by striking, laughing at, or ignoring others. Allowing clients to "tell it like it is" is not the end of the process, however. The helping relationship should have purpose beyond relating unpleasant feelings. If solutions are not sought, talking will serve only to frustrate clients further.

A distinction should be made between thinking *about* a problem and thinking *through* a problem. In the first instance little more than free association of ideas takes place. In the second instance more purposeful things occur: A problem is acknowledged; its implications are examined; solutions are contemplated. Thinking through a problem is physically as well as mentally stimulating. The heart beats faster, and perspiration may break out. The whole person gets caught up in thinking through a problem. Helpers must not push clients to hurry this process. The helper who chides a client, "If you really wanted to, you would make the necessary adjustments" is insensitive to the complexities of problem identification and altering established behavior.

3. *Clients who want to change may not know how or may feel threatened by the thought of changing.* Some persons with disabilities become obsessed with the fear that they will be publicly embarrassed or lose what little secruity they have if they behave differently. They know how to behave as cripples but are unsure what will

happen to them if they stop playing the role of helpless, dependent persons. Some families structure their lives around taking care of members with disabilities. There is no denying the vulnerability inherent in trying new behavior. When persons with disabilities expose themselves this way, they may indeed lose something.

4. *It is imperative that helpers focus on problems they can help clients think through.* Helpers should do the job they are paid to do: focus on the problems their job description implies or delineates. It is helpful to focus on immediate crisis situations or the single most important issue at the moment but not to become a participant in a client's flight. Experienced helpers know when and where to refer clients when they are unable to deal with them.

REFERENCES

Boyd, Malcolm. *Human Like Me, Jesus.* New York: Simon & Schuster, 1971.

Buber, Martin. *Pointing the Way.* New York: Harper & Row, 1957.

Carkhuff, Robert R. *Helping and Human Relations: Vol. 1. Selections and Training.* New York: Holt, Rinehart & Winston, 1969.

Hall, Edward T. *The Silent Language.* New York: Doubleday, 1959.

Harding, M. Esther. *The "I" and the "Not-I."* Princeton, NJ: Princeton University Press, 1965.

Kierkegaard, Søren. *The Works of Love.* New York: Harper & Row, 1962.

Maslow, Abraham. *Motivation and Personality.* New York: Harper & Row, 1970.

Maslow, Abraham H. *The Farther Reaches of Human Nature.* New York: Viking Press, 1971.

Menninger, Karl. *Love Against Hate.* New York: Harcourt, Brace & World, 1942.

Perlman, Helen Harris. *Social Casework: A Problem-Solving Process.* Chicago: University of Chicago Press, 1957.

Tournier, Paul. *The Meaning of Persons.* New York: Harper & Row, 1957.

Storr, Anthony. *The Integrity of Personality.* New York: Atheneum, 1961.

Additional Readings

Barsch, Ray H. *The Parents of the Handicapped Child.* Springfield, IL: Charles C Thomas, 1968.

Blondis, Marion N., and Jackson, Barbara E. *Nonverbal Communication with Patients: Back to the Human Touch.* Somerset, NJ: John Wiley & Sons, 1982.

Bowe, Frank. *Rehabilitating America Toward Independence for Disabled and Elderly People.* New York: Harper & Row, 1980.

Howard, William L., Dardig, Jill C., and Rossett, Allison. *Working with Parents of*

Handicapped Children. Columbus, OH: Charles E. Merrill, 1979.

Hull, Kent. *The Rights of Physically Handicapped People: An American Civil Liberties Unit Handbook.* New York: Avon Books, 1979.

Lindemann, James E. *Psychological and Behavioral Aspects of Physical Disability: A Manual for Health Practioners.* New York: Plenum Press, 1981.

Luterman, David. *Counseling Parents of Hearing-impaired Children.* Boston: Little, Brown, 1979.

Noland, Robert. *Counseling Parents of the Ill and the Handicapped.* Springfield, IL: Charles C Thomas, 1979.

Raphael, Alan J., Karpt, David A., and Sills, Frances W. Human relations training program: Prescription for rehab staff satisfaction. *Rehab Lit, 41*:16–18, 1980.

Ross, Ruth-Ellen K. *Handicapped People in Society: Ideas and Activities for Teachers.* Morristown, NJ: Silver Burdett, 1981.

Roessler, Richard T., and Rubin, Stanford E. *Case Management and Rehabilitation Counseling: Procedures and Techniques.* Baltimore: University Park Press, 1982.

Spiegal, Allen D., and Podair, Simon. *Rehabilitating People with Disabilities into the Mainstream of Society.* Park Ridge, NJ: Noyes Medical, 1981.

Vash, Carolyn L. *The Psychology of Disability.* New York: Springer, 1981.

Webster, Elizabeth J. (Ed.). *Professional Approaches to Parents of Handicapped Children.* Springfield, IL: Charles C Thomas, 1976.

Wright, George N. *Total Rehabilitation.* Boston: Little, Brown, 1980.

Chapter 11

TIPS FOR PEOPLE WITH DISABILITIES

Laugh and the world laughs with you, cry and you cry alone"
is an old saying that describes two reactions to problem-solving
behaviors. The authors are not suggesting that people should
take their disabilities lightly, because being disabled is a serious
matter. However, they are suggesting that instead of viewing
a disability as an end to life, it is much more productive to view it
as an aspect of living. This is a proactive, as opposed to a reactive,
approach to disabilities. It is true that crying over one's disability
is likely to generate sympathy, but feelings of sorrow and pity soon
give way to antagonism or indifference, especially when individuals do little to overcome their impairments. Sadness is not a solid
foundation upon which to build relationships.

Similar to a child who feels anger and temporary hatred for his
mother following an argument, persons with disabilities often
experience feelings of guilt, self-consciousness, inadequacy, depression, and shame following behavior to elicit sympathy. Persons without disabilities tend to send out mixed messages with
regard to their feelings about the situation, and their interaction
becomes less helpful. On the one hand, they may treat people with
disabilities as dependent persons who do not have the full range of
feelings, emotions, wants, and responsibilities of able-bodied people.
On the other hand, they may send signals that say to people with
disabilities that they should feel good about themselves because,
despite their physical limitations, they are worthwhile human
beings. These mixed messages confuse and greatly affect both
parties.

FEELINGS

No matter how positive the self-image of persons with disabilities, there will be times when they will feel inadequate. These negative feelings may be partially due to their disability and partially due to the fact that all people periodically have doldrums. This is normal behavior. Too often, people with disabilities are made to feel guilty because they become unhappy with their lives. Books and articles written by "experts" frequently chide people with disabilities for being human. When one takes a careful look at what these authors are saying, it is a message of Spartan self-discipline. This regimen is not realistic, and it most certainly is not achievable.

A person with a disability should not believe that he or she is emotionally ill if there are times when feelings of inferiority and shame, to mention just two, take hold. It is not easy living in a human fishbowl; persons staring or making comments about an individual's disability draw attention to his or her limitations. It is not abnormal or a sign of emotional instability to react negatively to being the object of attention, but it is abnormal to spend an inordinate amount of time feeling inferior or ashamed. Many individuals with disabilities forget that *all* humans, regardless of their physical condition, experience these feelings. For example, an able-bodied male who is in good physical condition may feel inferior when he sees a person with a physique that in his estimation is more developed than his own. The same is true for a female who observes another female who she thinks is better looking. There will always be someone with more or fewer attributes that a person values, and individuals who compete to be number one run the risk of losing self-esteem.

The authors' message to persons with disabilities is this: "Do not think that because of your disability your life must be considerably different than that of other people." They acknowledge and have discussed in previous chapters that a disability imposes limitations that may require special attention. However, at the other end of the continuum—and equally wrong—is the idea that an individual has to be Mr. or Ms. Superdisabled in order to be accepted. On the contrary, people with disabilities are entitled to be as average as people without disabilities. Not only are they entitled, but in reality they are.

More important than trying to excel in all behaviors is the need to express the broad range of feelings and emotions, as long as an individual abides by moral, social, and legal standards that restrict infringement on the rights of others. At this point, it is important to repeat what has been stated in previous chapters: A physical disability should neither restrict an individual from expressing himself or herself nor be a license to abuse others. A brief discussion of the stages of development and expression of feelings and social competence follows.

SOCIAL DEVELOPMENT

Information about child development has accumulated so rapidly that it is now subdivided into intellectual, physical, emotional, and social areas of research. This separation does not negate the fact that no one phase of development takes place independently of the others. For example, physical impairments frequently interfere with school adjustment; the effective use of language is closely related to social relationships; emotionally disturbed children are not likely to do well in school; and acceptance by the peer group is an important factor in a child's success in school. There are many ways to tell if a person with a disability is having growth problems, including observing the stages and periods listed below.

Certain motor behavior patterns are common in all children. Experimental evidence indicates that physical maturation determines the rate and pattern of mental growth. Little skill has developed until the child has matured sufficiently to engage in a particular activity, and each child's developmental pattern is unique. The internal growth process of the body organs and functions is called *maturation*. Specific organs do not function until minimum growth has taken place. For example, a sighted child does not learn to read until his or her nervous system has developed sufficiently for language capacity, eye control, and ability to concentrate. Obviously, eye control is not a factor in blind children learning to read Braille.

The age at which children are ready to read and write is determined by their level of development—neuromuscular, physical, and intellectual—and by their earlier experiences. Children with physical and social disabilities tend to be slower in learning to read and write, but all children tend to move in their learning from concrete to abstract. Therefore children who have disabilities should be actively involved with materials, substances, tools, and concrete situations.

Jean Piaget (1954) demonstrated that the very young child is easily and quickly confused by apparent changes in sizes and objects. Preschool children have not yet learned some of the basic physical constants of their environment. That is, they do not know that the weight, volume, length, and quantity of objects remain constant despite changes in their shapes or the contexts in which they appear. Thus, a two-year-old will acknowledge that two identical glasses contain the same amount of milk, but if the contents of one glass are emptied into a taller glass, he is likely to decide that the taller glass has more milk. His understanding of the concept is not yet stable and abstract.

Jerome Bruner (1966) emphasized four factors related to maturation: Linguistic skills are best taught at an early age; mental growth is based not on gradual increases of associations or stimulus-response connections but rather on sudden sharp rises and stops as certain capacities develop; children are in a state of readiness at an earlier age than previously had been thought; and the emphasis in education should be on skills and areas related to learning skills, with a curriculum based on self-reward sequences.

Although social development begins slowly at birth, it is greatly accelerated during the preschool and elementary school years when a child's interaction with peers becomes more frequent and intense. As preschool children grow older, demands for socialization cause them to spend less time in nonsocial, individualistic activities. They gradually learn to repress egocentric behaviors in favor of group-approved responses. The sociopsychological processes of interaction through which the individual learns the habits, beliefs, values, and skills for effective group participation is called *socialization.* The stages or periods of socialization are overlapping. The major function of socialization is to transform an untrained human organism into an effective member of a society. The most important elements of socialization take place during childhood, but growth is lifelong.

Growing up is synonymous with developing appropriate skills, knowledge, feelings, and attitudes. As children's physical and psychological capacities develop, they are confronted with new societal expectations and norms. The cultural pressures for conformity are difficult for children without disabilities and almost impossible for those who have them. Common developmental tasks range from learning sex-appropriate behavior to becoming socially responsible.

Robert Havighurst (1953) suggested the following list of developmental tasks:

- *Early childhood*—learning to walk; learning to take solid foods; learning to control the elimination of body wastes; learning sex differences and sexual modesty, learning physiological stability; forming simple concepts of social and physical reality; learning to relate oneself emotionally to parents, siblings, and other people; and learning to distinguish right from wrong
- *Middle childhood*—learning physical skills necessary for ordinary games; building a wholesome self-concept; learning to get along with age-mates; developing fundamental skills in reading, writing, and calculating; developing concepts necessary for everyday living; developing conscience, morality, and a scale of values; achieving personal independence; and developing attitudes toward social groups and institutions
- *Adolescence*—achieving more mature relations with age-mates; achieving a masculine or feminine social identity; accepting one's physique and using the body effectively; achieving independence of parents and other adults; selecting and preparing for an occupation; preparing for marriage and family life; developing intellectual skills and concepts necessary for civic competence; desiring and achieving socially responsible behavior; and acquiring a set of values and an ethical system
- *Early adulthood*—selecting a mate; learning to live with a marriage partner; starting a family; rearing children; manag-

ing a home; getting started in an occupation; taking on civic responsibility; and finding a congenial social group

- *Middle age*—achieving adult civic responsibility; establishing and maintaining an economic standard of living; assisting teenage children to become responsible adults; developing adult leisure-time activities; relating oneself to one's spouse as a person; accepting and adjusting to the physiological changes of middle age; and adjusting to aging parents
- *Later maturity*—adjusting to decreasing physical strength and health; adjusting to retirement and reduced income; adjusting to the death of one's spouse; establishing an explicit affiliation with one's age-group; meeting social and civic obligations; and establishing satisfactory physical living arrangements

Erik Erikson (1950) delineated eight stages in the life cycle:

- *Trust vs. mistrust* (*birth to one year*)—If children's basic needs are met, they will think the world is a safe and dependable place. If their basic needs are not met or if they are inconsistently met, they will define the world as a place of fear and suspicion.
- *Autonomy vs. doubt* (*two to three years*)—If children are encouraged to do things they are capable of doing, at their own pace and in their own time, they learn autonomy. If they are encouraged to do too many things—things they don't want to do or things they can't do—they doubt their ability to deal with the environment.
- *Initiative vs. guilt* (*four to five years*)—If children are allowed to initiate activities and if parents take time to answer their questions, they will not be afraid to tackle new things. If their movements are greatly restricted and they are made to feel that their questions are unimportant, they will feel guilty doing things on their own.
- *Industry vs. inferiority* (*six to eleven years*)—If children are encouraged to make and do things, are allowed to finish what they start, and are praised for the efforts and results, they become industrious. If they are ridiculed or ignored for trying to do things, they feel inferior.
- *Identity vs. role confusion* (*twelve to eighteen years*)—If adoles-

cents succeed in integrating roles in different situations and also experience continuity in their perceptions of self, they develop a positive self-identity. If they are unable to establish a sense of stability in the various roles they play, then confusion results.

- *Intimacy vs. isolation* (*young adulthood*) — This stage is characterized by being pulled to identify with others and, conversely, being repelled by them because of competitive, combative relations.
- *Generalivity vs. self-absorption* (*middle age*) — This is the struggle between establishing and guiding the next generation and being a victims of one's own self-concerns.
- *Integrity vs. despair* (*old age*) — Integrity is acceptance of one's life cycle as something that had to be, while despair is the feeling that time has run out to try alternative roads to integrity.

Piaget (1952) described four stages or periods of intellectual development:

- *Sensorimotor* (*birth to two years*) — This stage is characterized by learning about properties of things through the senses and motor activity. This leads to new ways of handling situations.
- *Preoperational* (*two to seven years*) — By learning symbols, children are able to manipulate symbols and objects mentally. This also allows acquisition of language that is egocentric; words have a unique meaning to each child. Gradually the child learns to think of more than one quality at a time and to understand conversation.
- *Concrete operational* (*seven to eleven years*) — The child learns to manipulate mentally concrete experiences that earlier had to be manipulated physically; the child develops the ability to deal with operations but not to generalize beyond his or her actual experiences.
- *Formal operational* (*eleven years and older*) — The child develops the ability to deal with things not present and with abstractions.

Drawing on Piaget's work, Bruner (1962) identified three stages of concept development. During the first stage, *preoperational*, which generally ends at about age five or six, the child is concerned with manipulating objects on a trial-and-error basis. During the second stage, *concrete operations*, which begins after the child enters school, the ability to organize data through contact with concrete objects emerges, and the child learns to use organized data in the solution of problems. During the third stage, *formal operations*, which usually begins between the ages of ten and fourteen, the child acquires the ability to operate on hypothetical propositions without having the concrete objects visible.

Childhood

The average child's physical growth is as rapid from birth to five years of age as it is from six to sixteen. During the first five years, depending on the disability and parental reaction, a child with a disability may grow from a helpless, dependent infant to an active pseudo-independent person. Of course, if parents are overprotective, the child remains helpless and dependent. For most preschool children, the large muscles mature rapidly but are not under complete control.

During childhood, social conflicts tend to decrease, and friendly interactions increase. The patterns of friendship change markedly with age changes. For example, between the ages of two and three the number of friends increases; after this time the major change is in the closeness of attachment to a few friends. Varying modes of popularity and leadership emerge. By the time they reach kindergarten, most children have a fairly definite idea of other children with whom they would like to play. Some children with disabilities are constantly sought out by other children for playmates; others are rejected and avoided. A few children with disabilities assume leadership roles; most are content to be followers. On the whole, the interactions of preschool children are characterized by cooperation and friendship.

Unlike preschool friendships, which are casual and transient, elementary school relationships become more intense and lasting. With the exception of their parents and a few teachers, elementary schoolchildren's closest friends are their age-mates.

MIDDLE CHILDHOOD (ages six through twelve) is dominated by "gang" activities. The growth of bones, muscles, and nervous tissue is dramatic during this period. The long bones of the legs and arms grow rapidly, and this gives most children a tall, thin look, as contrasted with their previous short, stocky appearance. Along with the rapid development of the large muscles of the legs, back, shoulders, arms, and wrist comes an increase in physical activity. Physically immobile and slow children are left behind. This is especially true for children with impaired muscles and nervous tissue.

The nervous system reaches its maximum rate of development around ten years of age, and at twelve the brain has reached its maximum size. This results in a higher level of intellectual development than of muscular dexterity. Thus, a miniature adult is trapped in a child's body. The quest for redefinition begins. Sexual differences are learned and internalized. So, too, is the need to challenge authority.

PREADOLESCENCE OR PUBERTY (ages ten through twelve) is characterized by many conditions, including a growth spurt, awakening sexuality, and an increase in peer group relationships. Except for infancy, the body undergoes the most rapid changes in size and shape during this period. Children aged ten, eleven, and twelve begin to "look down on" little children and underdeveloped age-mates. (Persons with physical disabilities are disproportionately represented in the latter category.) Along with these changes, the reproductive system starts to mature, causing sex-linked physical characteristics to appear: Girls develop obvious breasts and begin to produce feminine hormones; boys get more muscular and begin to produce masculine hormones. This is hardly the period of "latency" that early psychologists imagined it to be. Skin blemishes and increased weight add to the awkwardness of this period.

During this period, friends tend to resemble each other in social class, chronological age, physical maturity, and ethnic identity. This, without much doubt, is one of the most difficult periods for socially rejected children with disabilities. Negative attitudes that children have toward disabilities are reinforced, and positive ones are questioned during the pairing off for dates. This also is the time when positive contacts with persons with disabilities can alter prejudicial attitudes. As a group, it is accurate to say, all preadolescents are characterized by prolonged depressed and negativistic states.

The social meanings of their disabilities are learned by most children mainly from interaction with their significant others. Overprotection by parents and siblings provides the child with a disability with his or her first debilitating concept: "I am fragile. I am not expected to do the same things as able-bodied children. I am not responsible for my behavior." This attitude does not prepare children for interacting with age-mates as equals, but it does prepare them for rejection. One of the most devastating realities many children with disabilities experience in childhood is rejection. Consistently being the last person chosen in team sports and being excluded from group conversations and peer activities are demoralizing to young developing egos—and older ones, too.

Children with disabilities tend to develop behaviors to protect their egos from constant rebuffing. Isolation and hostility are only two of the protective behaviors that children with disabilities may exhibit. Sitting in the back of the classroom and not participating in class discussion are early signs of isolation. Becoming a bully and responding defensively to teachers, parents, and other authority figures are not always signs of tough kids. Often these behaviors mask fragile and frustrated lives: Limiting association with people lessens the chances of being rejected by them. The child with a disability may view this behavior as the best way of dealing with his or her frustration. In reality this may be the only way he or she knows to react.

It may be painful for children with disabilities to tell others about the frustration they experience trying to fit in with "normal" people. However, this problem can be effectively dealt with only by sharing it with caring people and devising appropriate coping mechanisms. Teachers usually are good listeners, and most parents care about the welfare of their children and are interested in such problems. If adults are not acceptable, most children have at least one close friend with whom they can share intimate feelings. Although problems centering on disabilities can be discussed with friends, it is wise to remember that whether or not friends have disabilities they also have problems, and care must be taken not to "dump" a load of problems on them.

Adolescence

The period from puberty to the late teens or early twenties is adolescence. Many of the problems described earlier are carried over into this period, often described as the "impossible period" between childhood and adulthood. Thus, there are fears centering on physical appearance, sex, social status, and vocation. Being denied many of the rights of either children or adults, they are nevertheless expected to fulfill many of the obligations of both groups. That is, they are expected to remain obedient to their parents, to control their sex impulses, to select a vocation, and otherwise to begin to act as adults.

This is a period in which young people need association with the opposite sex; they also need to evolve their own theory of life. Dating becomes a central concern for both sexes. Along with the problem of getting dates come issues centering on the outer limits of heterosexual and homosexual relationships. In general, adolescent girls engage in less premarital sexual intercourse than boys, but standards of acceptable sexual behavior vary with social class. For example, studies indicate that masturbation is quite widely practiced among middle-class children, whereas sexual intercourse is much more frequent among lower-class children. Because of their more limited opportunities to engage in dating activities, adolescents with physical disabilities, moreso than other adolescents, are likely to masturbate than to engage in sexual intercourse.

Adolescents identify most strongly with their own peers and form cliques. Members of cliques usually come from the same racial and socioeconomic backgrounds and therefore have much the same interests and values. Cliques are dominant forces because they are based on personal compatibility, congeniality, and mutual admiration. If members of cliques are conscious of their physical appearance, youths with obvious physical impairments are excluded.

Most adolescent groups reinforce and strengthen the values that members have acquired from their parents. In other words, peer groups are less originators than reinforcers of values and behaviors developed in the family. This includes values and behaviors pertaining to people with disabilities. However, in some areas such as dress, music, and slang, peer groups aid adolescents in achieving independence from adults. By sticking together and behaving alike, they are able to insulate themselves from outside pressures to conform to all adult norms and behaviors.

Contrary to some opinions, most adolescents do not view their parents as unnecessary authoritarians. Instead, they consider them as necessary teachers of moral and ethical values. Thus, most adolescents grow up and behave like their parents. Muzafer and Carolyn Sherif (1964) clearly demonstrated the extent to which all adolescents are affected by middle-class values:

> There is one clear and striking generalization about the high school youth which holds in all areas and despite their differing backgrounds: Their values and goals earmark all as youth exposed to the American ideology of success and wanting the tangible symbols of that success. There were no differences between the youth in different areas with respect to desires for material goods. In addition to comfortable housing, the symbols of success for these adolescents include a car in every garage, a telephone, television set, transitor radio, fashionable clothing, time to enjoy them, and money to provide them. [p. 199]

Little has changed since the Sherifs conducted their studies.

This period is especially trying for youths with disabilities who begin serioulsy to question their future: "Will I get married?" "Will I have children?" "If I have children will they be disabled?" "Will my children be ashamed of me?" "Will I be able to find a job?" These are but a few of the future-oriented questions that nag disabled adolescents. All of these are valid questions that must be dealt with in a caring manner. Failure to do so will only add to the moodiness, confusion, and oversensitivity that characterize adolescents. Unfortunately, most adolescents with disabilities are afraid and ashamed to ask adults these questions. They need to know that some of these questions, particularly those pertaining to marriage, are of concern to children who do not have disabilities.

Adulthood

Depending on the source consulted, adulthood begins at age eighteen, nineteen, twenty, or twenty-one. In some communities, adolescents are physically and psychologically adults but legally classified as juveniles. Conversely, many persons are adults legally but psychologically less mature than adolescents. Generally, *young adulthood,* up to the age of forty, is a period of great mobility and transition. Most young adults move from economic dependence on parents to self-support, from being at home to starting their own homes. They engage in a variety of jobs and experiment with different life-styles. These changes are more difficult and less likely for those with disabilities, who frequently are neither encouraged nor allowed to grow up.

The period of *middle age* (from about forty to sixty-five years of age) is characterized by depression, restlessness, irritability, anxiety, and physiological upheaval. Concern about health and physical appearance is increased during the middle years. Consequently, exercise and diets are ritualistically followed. For individuals with disabilities who have been able to secure steady employment during their young adulthood, middle age is a period of economic security and relative comfort. This also is the time when most people realize that they are unlikely to attain many of their childhood dreams of success. For some persons this leads to prolonged disillusionment; for others it leads to contentment with what they have been able to achieve. For persons with permanent disabilities, this is a time to accept their condition or lapse into continual depression.

The period of *old age* starts at about sixty-five years of age. Old age is a great equalizer for individuals who acquired physical disabilities during their younger years. Physical deterioration and chronic disabilities and diseases become prevalent for all people during old age. Physiologically, the body begins to break down, and, psychologically, the mind becomes less proficient. It is during old age that most people become concerned about disabling conditions. Often, their concern is too little, too late. Their fate, like that of many persons with disabilities of all ages, is social disengagement and alienation. Fortunately, conditions are changing for young persons with disabilities and the aged. Gradually, Americans are beginning to fashion out productive lives during disability and old age.

The rest of the authors' comments are directed to people with disabilities. While directed to them, these remarks may be helpful to other persons who find themselves in teaching, counseling, rehabilitation, and other helping roles.

SELF-ACCEPTANCE

No matter what age a person is, it is important that he or she know and accept himself or herself. The person who has a positive self-concept and strong self-acceptance will do more than survive. He or she will flourish as a person. It is difficult to convince other people to accept one, however, if one does not accept oneself. Part of the self-identity of a person with a disability is the disability. The person who has a strong sense of self-acceptance is not afraid to acknowledge his or her disability, nor is he or she afraid to admit strengths and weaknesses or to be rejected by individuals who do not like disabilities. He or she does not waste energies being negative and defensive but instead uses them for positive, creative activities and interactions. The individual who has not learned to accept his or her disability becomes a negative prophecy that fulfills itself.

People with disabilities should accept their disability as a fact of life but not as their whole life. In other words, they should view the disability and its limitations as a reality, but their entire life should not be controlled by it. To be consumed by their disability will not allow the development of their strengths and positive potentials; instead, almost all of their energies—mental, physical, and emotional—will be drained in an attempt to "live with a physical disability." Few people are fortunate enough to learn to accept themselves totally. All people fall short of perfection in almost all matters; all do things that cause them to dislike themselves. This is normal. However, some persons dislike themselves most of the time. That is not normal. They must learn that because they are not able to do some things with the style, grace, or quickness of persons without disabilities, this is not failure. On the contrary, it is *difference*.

People tend to respond to others in ways that reflect how they

regard themselves. Self-assured persons do not have to use others
to build their own egos. They give freely of themselves and have
no need to put others down. Individuals who have low self-
acceptance use people to support their own ego but give little to
them in return. They are immature and unable to tolerate situations that do not support them. Often they project onto others
aspects of themselves that they find despicable. If one is a mature
person, one will not have to find scapegoats for one's own inadequacies. Instead, one will seek self-improvement.

The self-assured disabled person mixes well with other people,
and this, in turn, enhances his or her self-esteem. The person who
has a low self-concept avoids people or, at the other extreme,
displays destructive, competitive, defensive, or dependent behavior.
This latter behavior repels friends and irritates enemies. This sets
up a no-win situation.

POSITIVE THOUGHTS

An acquaintance of one of the authors decided to establish a
business. In the initial planning stage, he talked with many people
who had attempted to establish a similar business but had failed.
His idea was to learn as many of their mistakes as possible so that
he could avoid making them in his own business. Approximately
one year after the establishment of his business, the young entre-
preneur declared bankruptcy. Part of the reason for his failure was
that he had, without realizing what he was doing, programmed
himself to think negatively. He became so obsessed with the ways
his business could fail that he forgot to think of the many ways to
make it succeed.

Several books focusing on positive thinking have been written,
and the authors of some of these books make comfortable livings
teaching the "power of positive thinking." The main theme running through most discussions of positive thinking is "Believe in
yourself." Although societal attitudes get in the way of the self-
actualization of people with disabilities, the major obstacle often
is the people themselves. Too many persons with disabilities allow
themselves to think negatively. If a person believes that he or she

cannot make a positive contribution to society, it is very likely that he or she will not.

REALISM

Realistic ideas of one's abilities and limitations are prerequisites to being a successful person. To attempt to accomplish what may seem to be the impossible is not foolish. In fact, many great accomplishments, such as Orville and Wilbur Wright's maiden flight at Kitty Hawk, North Carolina, Henry Ford's horseless carriage, and the development of television, were at one time considered impossible feats. However, continually attempting to accomplish things that have been proven to be beyond one's capabilities is foolish expenditure of one's energies. As has been discussed in previous chapters, everyone has limitations, and the key is to become successful in doing the possible. One must recognize and accept one's limitations as well as identify one's strengths and build on them.

Too often, people with disabilities feel that they must become superdisabled in order to be recognized as worthy human beings. In the process of becoming superdisabled they forget to be human. Stated another way, some persons devote so much energy and time to trying to be superstars that they become subnormal failures. They fail to develop into well-rounded individuals who can function in many social and economic settings. They should take inventory of their skills, determining what they do well and also what they do poorly. They should not hesitate to participate in activities in which they are average performers. Most people will have skills similar to theirs; therefore, they will fit in. If people participate only in activities in which they are the best, friends will avoid them, because no one likes to feel inferior. People should not avoid those things in which they perform poorly; to do so will cause them to miss opportunities to improve their skills. However, they should not subject themselves to humiliation by constantly trying to do things that are virtually impossible for them to accomplish with any degree of skill and success.

RESPONSIBILITY

A physical disability is no reason for a person to surrender his or her life to others. Regardless of how caring, empathic, and sincere a helper is, the person with a disability is the best person to control his or her own life. Hospitalization, physical restoration, personal adjustment counseling, vocational evaluation, vocational counseling, and job placement create opportunities for independence or dependence. Too much attention and too much care can create a feeling of helplessness. The severity of the limitations imposed by a disability obviously affects the degree of independence one may have. However, dependency should not mean total loss of control over decision making. Even individuals with severe disabilities can exercise some control over their lives. Decisions such as what to eat within their diet, what to watch on television, or which book to read can be made by most concerned persons.

It is easy for people to blame others for their own mistakes or problems. In fact, it is psychologically more satisfying to think that others are the cause of a behavior, especially if that behavior is not to their liking. However, personal growth begins when people accept responsibility for their behavior. Becoming a responsible person is not always easy. Being responsible for oneself is a demanding task. Although people have certain basic needs from birth to death, which, if left unmet, cause them to suffer, they are not naturally endowed with the ability to fulfill them. If the ability to satisfy basic needs were as much a part of people as are the needs themselves, they would not have any psychosocial problems. Being responsible for oneself often is easier said than done.

EFFECTIVE COMMUNICATION

One of the most effective ways of determining one's own destiny is to communicate effectively with others. Effective communication means that one will—

1. *understand the roles* of each player in the drama of the helping relationship. It usually is quite obvious what the role of the person with the disability is to be: He or she becomes an individ-

ual to be helped, to be rehabilitated, to be evaluated. However, in contrast to the role of the client, the role of the helper is not always clear. Questions that a client must ask are "What do you do?" "What kind of help can you provide me?" "What do you expect of me?" "What are your limits?" In other words, "Where does your role end and another helper's role begin?" Once the client has answers to these questions, he or she can effectively interact with helpers. Without answers to these questions, the client will not know what to expect in the helping relationship and should refuse to commit himself or herself to unknown people.

2. *listen to what others say.* Although total silence is not recommended in the interaction with a helper, neither is nonstop talking recommended. Talking is one way of relieving anxiety, but excessive talking creates anxiety in the person to whom one is speaking. Effective listening requires paying careful attention to not only the spoken words but also the speaker's body language. If a client is sighted, he or she may obtain a great deal of information by observing the helper's facial expressions and body movement. If the client is blind but not deaf, he or she should pay attention to how the helper talks, i.e. inflections and pauses.

3. *organize one's thoughts* and make sense of the many perceptions running through one's mind. Some of these thoughts may be: "I am uncomfortable with what he is saying." "She is asking me to do something I am afraid to do." "That is not what I want to do." "What will my friends think of this?" "I will be embarrassed wearing that thing." "Will my family accept me?" It is imperative that the client learn to sort out and deal with the disquieting feelings of the moment and carefully discuss them with a helper. It is not uncommon when under stress to jump from one subject to another. Therefore, it is helpful to state feelings and make points clearly and coherently.

4. *wait for reaction* once something has been presented to the helper. This is more effective than skipping from one concern to another. Waiting for a reaction means more than listening to the words. It also means, where possible, observing the person's body reaction.

5. *keep an open mind.* This means more than being receptive to the helper's ideas. It means being willing to question the helper's

recommendations. Because an individual is a professional does not mean that he or she automatically knows what is best for a client. Besides, it is the client's life.

6. *make sure of the communication.* Once an agreement has been made regarding the subject under discussion, every attempt should be made to ensure that the client's understanding and the helper's understanding are the same. The best rehabilitation plans will crumble if all parties are not operating from the same reference points.

PRIDE

Many persons without disabilities find it difficult to imagine people with disabilities as being happy. Yet, many of them are happy. Physical wholeness does not bestow virtues, nor does a disability take them away. An individual can, paraphrasing black Americans, have a disability but feel beautiful and proud. By projecting an image of a proud person, the individual projects the image of a person not ashamed of himself or herself. Of course, there is truth in negative and positive images. Pride is created and projected to others when people with disabilities respect themselves and demand that others do likewise. This demand means that these individuals will not allow others to devalue their abilities by concentrating on their limitations. Pride comes from not devaluing oneself.

SELF-IMPROVEMENT

The self is always in a state of change; it is never a finished product. One will not be, nor should one expect to be, the same person tomorrow as today. People are always, in Gordon Allport's (1955) words, in the process of "becoming." However, each individual develops habits and defense mechanisms that slow the process of change. Consequently, it is difficult to make sweeping changes in personality.

Often people with disabilities try to improve their self-esteem through superficial changes such as prostheses, speech, clothing, and cosmetics. These efforts result in real self-improvement only when they accept their disabilities and change their own negative attitudes and behavior. The difficulty inherent in changing some low self-concepts is that they are too deeply rooted in attitudes and defenses that do not give in easily to do-it-yourself approaches. In these instances, professional helpers are needed to facilitate the change process. This help may come in individual or group therapy situations.

Self-help groups for persons with disabilities are springing up all over the world. In many instances they are highly successful in treating individuals who for various reasons have turned to lay persons, rather than professionals, for help. The spirit of commitment and fellowship is very high in most of these organizations. Under no circumstances should anyone discount the importance or effectiveness of well-conceived self-help groups. Each individual must determine whether any of them can be helpful to him or her. For many persons and their families, these groups are vital in the rehabilitation process. There is more, not less, cooperation between professionals and self-help groups.

SUMMARY

If a person is to engage successfully in self-improvement, he or she must, as pointed out earlier, first assess strengths and weaknesses to get a clear understanding of what he or she is and would like to become. Being honest about what one sees in the mirror of life can be unnerving. One may see ugliness and weakness in oneself that one deplores. It is seldom painless to view oneself in an objective, detached manner. Most people need help in taking off their rose-colored glasses, and almost all people need help when they try to correct what they do not like about themselves. Self-improvement is a difficult process, but it is achievable. The hallmarks of a person with a disability who is capable of successful self-improvement are honesty, tenacity, and humility.

NOTE TO HELPERS

If helpers are to understand people with disabilities, they must first understand people. An individual with a disability is not an alien creature. W. Paul Torrance (1970) provided an interesting perspective on human behavior. The authors have modified his list of characteristics to fit people with disabilities:

1. "Wanting to know" — This is evident in the curiosity of persons with disabilities who ask questions, become absorbed in the search for the truth of their disabilities, try to make sense out of their world, make guesses and test them, and try to discover their limits and the limits of their conditions. *Helpers must help them to know.*

2. "Digging deeper" — The genuinely human person with a disability is not satisfied with quick, easy, superficial answers. *Helpers must not give such answers.*

3. "Looking twice and listening for smells" — The person with a disability can never be satisfied with his or her situation by looking at it from an intellectual distance or seeing a report or hearing the helper's words or touching equipment. He or she will want to get to know it from different angles, perspectives, and senses. It is not necessarily a sign of distrust when a client tries to find out things on his or her own terms. *Helpers must realize that it is the client's life and let him or her have it.*

4. "Listening to a cat" — Too many helpers can neither talk to nor listen with understanding to a cat. Much human communication is nonverbal. In the helping process, words usually are insufficient for communicating the deepest and most genuine concerns of one person for another. *Helpers must learn to communicate nonverbally and to understand nonverbal communication.*

5. "Crossing out mistakes" — Persons with disabilities who try to achieve their potentialities inevitably make mistakes. They lose in humanness when they avoid doing difficult and worthwhile things because of the fear of failure. *Helpers must help them not to be afraid to try new things and must not punish or ridicule them if they fail.*

6. *"Getting into and out of deep water"* — Testing the limits of one's skills and abilities, disability, and personal resources means taking calculated risks. It means asking questions for which no ready answers exist. *An effective helper assists clients to sort out possible alternatives.*

7. "Having a ball" — To be truly human is to be able to laugh,

play, fantasy, and loaf. *Helpers should encourage their clients to take time out to relax.*

8. "Cutting a hole to see through"—This is a tolerance for complexity. By opening up the windows of their lives, persons with disabilities see more of themselves. *An effective helper must be a window through which clients can gain a better understanding of the world beyond themselves.*

9. "Building sand castles"—In order to build a sand castle, one must be able to see sand not only as it is but also as it might be. To move from dependency to independence requires persons with disabilities to see their existence as it might be. *Helpers must encourage clients to plan and strive for their dreams but to do so in terms of the materials and resources they can realistically draw upon.*

10. "Singing in your own key"—Thoreau stated this idea very poetically: "If a man does not keep pace with his companions, perhaps it is because he hears a different drummer. Let him step to the music he hears, however measured or far away. It is not important that he matures as an apple tree or an oak. Shall he turn his spring into summer . . . ?" *Helpers should let their clients know that it is all right to do things differently, to be out of step with persons who do not have a disability.*

11. "Plugging in the sun"—For most persons with disabilities, the source of their energy comes from self-help groups and organizations that focus on the needs of persons with disabilities. *An effective helper learns the names and locations of local or regional organizations that pertain to people with disabilities.*

12. "Shaking hands with the future"—Becoming human means growing up or realizing yesterday's dreams and also creating new dreams. *Helpers must be willing to become their client's past, to terminate the helper-client relationship when their client has achieved his or her rehabilitation goals.*

Professional helpers must learn as much as they can about their clients and use this information to help make their rehabilitation as successful as possible. First, however, helpers must be willing to let their clients become whatever they become.

REFERENCES

Allport, Gordon W. *Becoming: Basic Considerations for a Psychology of Personality.* New Haven, CT: Yale University Press, 1955.

Bruner, Jerome S. *The Process of Education.* Cambridge, MA: Harvard University Press, 1962.

Bruner, Jerome S. *Toward a Theory of Instruction.* New York: Belknap, 1966.

Erikson, Erik H. *Children and Society.* New York: W. W. Norton, 1950.

Havinghurst, Robert J. *Human Development and Education.* New York: Longmans, Green, 1953.

Piaget, Jean. *The Language and Thought of the Child.* London: Routledge & Kegan Paul, 1952.

Piaget, Jean. *The Construction of Reality for the Child.* New York: Basic Books, 1954.

Sherif, Muzafer, and Sherif, Carolyn W. *Reference Groups.* New York: Harper & Row, 1964.

Torrance, W. Paul. What it means to be human. In Scobey, Mary-Margaret, and Graham, Grace (Eds.). *To Nurture Humanne: Commitment for the 70's.* Washington, DC: Association for Supervision and Curriculum Development, 1970.

Additional Readings

Alpiner, Jerome G. *Talk to Me: Vol. I: How Your Baby Grows and Vol. II: How to Help Your Baby.* Baltimore: Williams & Wilkins, 1977.

Atwater, Maxine H. *Rollin' On: A Wheelchair Guide to U.S. Cities.* New York: Dodd, Mead, 1978.

Ayrault, Evelyn West. *Sex, Love and the Physically Handicapped.* New York: Continuum, 1981.

Borman, Leonard D. (Ed.). *Helping People to Help Themselves: Self-Help and Prevention.* New York: Haworth Press, 1982.

Boshell, Buris R. *The Diabetic at Work and Play.* Springfield, IL: Charles C Thomas, 1979.

Bullard, David G., and Knight, Susan E. *Sexuality and Physical Disability: Personal Perspectives.* St. Louis: C. V. Mosby, 1981.

Burgdorf, Robert L. *The Legal Rights of Handicapped Persons: Cases, Materials and Texts.* Baltimore: Paul H. Brookes, 1980.

Christenson, Kathryn, and Miller, Kelvin. *Tributes to Courage.* Golden Valley, MN: Courage Center, 1980.

Cohen, Shirley. *Special People: A Brighter Future for Everyone with Physical, Mental and Emotional Disabilities.* Englewood Cliffs, NJ: Prentice-Hall, 1977.

Eisenberg, Myron G., Griggins, Cynthia, and Duval, Richard J. *Disabled People as Second-Class Citizens.* New York: Springer, 1982.

Forsythe, Elizabeth. *Living with Multiple Sclerosis.* Salem, NH: Faber & Faber, 1979.

Fraser, Malcolm. *Self-Therapy for the Stutterer.* Memphis, TN: Speech Foundation of America, 1982.

Gruen, Hannelore. *Self-Help for Patients with Arthritis.* Atlanta, GA: The Arthritis Foundation, 1980.

Hale, Glorya. *The Source Book for the Disabled: An Illustrated Guide for Easier and More Independent Living for Physically Disabled People, Their Families, and Friends.* New York: Paddington Press, 1979.

Howards, Irving. *Disability: From Social Problems to Federal Program.* New York: Praeger, 1980.

Hull, Kent. *The Rights of Physically Handicapped People: An American Civil Liberties Handbook.* New York: Avon Books, 1979.

Jay, Peggy. *Help Yourself: A Handbook for Hemiplegics and Their Families.* New York: State Mutual Book and Periodical Service, 1979.

Katz, Alfred H., and Knute, Martin. *A Handbook of Services for the Handicapped.* Westport, CT: Greenwood Press, 1982.

Lorig, Kate, and Fries, James F. *The Arthritis Helpbook: What You Can Do for Your Arthritis.* Reading, MA: Addison-Wesley, 1981.

Lunt, Suzanne. *A Handbook for the Disabled: Ideas and Innovations for Easier Living.* New York: Charles Scribner's Sons, 1982.

National Academy of Gallaudet College. *Living with Deaf-Blindness: Nine Profiles.* Washington, DC: National Academy, 1979.

Nichols, P. J. R. *Rehabilitation Medicine: The Management of Physical Disabilities.* Woburn, MA: Butterworth, 1980.

Office of Handicapped Individuals. *Directory of National Sources on Handicapping Conditions and Related Sources.* Washington, DC: Clearinghouse on the Handicapped, 1980.

Reamy, Lois. *Travel Ability: A Guide for Physically Disabled Travelers in the United States.* New York: Macmillan, 1978.

Robinault, Isabel P. *Sex, Society and the Disabled: A Developmental Inquiry into Roles, Reactions, and Responsibilities.* Hagerstown, MD: Harper & Row, 1978.

Rogers, Michael A. *Paraplegic: A Handbook of Practical Care and Advice.* Salem, NH: Faber & Faber, 1978.

Spradley, Thomas S., and Spradley, James P. *Deaf Like Me.* New York: Random House, 1978.

Ulene, Art, and Feldman, Sandy. *Help Yourself to Health: A Health Information and Services Directory.* New York: G. P. Putnam's Sons, 1980.

Volle, Frank O., and Heron, Patricia. *Epilepsy and You.* Springfield, IL: Charles C Thomas, 1978.

Chapter 12

FINAL THOUGHTS

Despite America's new national awareness of people with disabilities, there are still too few jobs for workers with disabilities, colleges and universities graduate few persons with permanent disabilities, and a disproportionate number of children with disabilities receive an inferior quality of public school education. In some ways, the conditions of people with disabilities are getting worse. Looking around their communities, they see too many persons with disabilities who are failures and too few who have made it into the mainstream. Similar environmental conditions have literally killed people of less fortitude; the price of survival is high. Often, people with disabilities are asked to forfeit their dignity. As the authors wrote this book, several threads of thought ran throughout the chapters. Briefly, some of them will be recast here into a mosaic of the forces impacting on and shaping the lives of the physically disabled.

HUMAN RIGHTS AND SURVIVAL

In 1948 the United Nations Declaration of Human Rights affirmed the "equal and inalienable rights of all members of the human family." Specifically concerning people with disabilities, this principle of human rights is applicable to their medical, psychological, and economic well-being. Accordingly, all persons with disabilities have the right to a standard of living adequate for the care of themselves and, where needed, their family, including food, shelter, clothing, and medical treatment. Unfortunately, most persons with disabilities are kept as consumers rather than given equal opportunity to be producers, and this prevents them from meeting their own needs.

Physical disability demoralizes, and one of the most insidious evils that accrues is that, historically, disability has been equated with laziness, inferiority, and lack of virtue. These epithets add humiliation to the other burdens of people who find themselves physically, emotionally, and/or socially disabled. Although there are ample religious admonitions concerning care for the disabled, many persons with the capability to assist often are remiss in their obligation mainly because they do not truly care about the disabled. To care is to believe that disabilities should not lead to loss of dignity, freedom, and security. It is easy to lose sight of the fact that people with disabilities, more so than others, are denied their rightful claim to equal opportunities and to global existence. Too often their success depends on the charity of others, and too often they are powerless by being passive and inactive citizens.

Even the major thrusts in medical science covertly and overtly define *people with disabilities* as undesirable. Consider the implications of deoxyribonucleic acid (DNA), called "the secret of life" by James Watson and Francis Crick, two Cambridge biologists, who discovered it in 1953. They ushered in the beginning of molecular biology. Add Herman Muller's program of genetic betterment, "germinal choice," with the techniques of artificial insemination and egg implantation. someday scientists may be able to clone "perfect" persons, *free of disabilities.*

Indeed, the baby factories of Aldous Huxley's *Brave New World* are already in progress. As they read science fiction and science facts, people with disabilities find little of themselves in the scenarios. There simply are no plans to reproduce disabilities. This fact is mentioned not to protest scientific advances but, instead, to illustrate why many people with disabilities react negatively to the quest for postmodern life forms. Until the medical revolution is finished, some babies will be born with disabilities, and some children and adults will become disabled, and they all will discover very few public signs that indicate they are wanted.

Also consider for a moment the possibility that most employers prefer robots over workers with disabilities not because they believe robots can do better work than these workers but because they believe robots *are* better. It can be argued that most workers act much like insufficient robots: They perform repetitive, mind-dulling tasks, ignore the deeper implications of their personal needs, and become sick in the process. It is much simpler to turn all work functions over to a machine. Indeed, automation tends to displace people with disabilities before it displaces the able-bodied. Yet, somehow those displaced defy social pressures, economic odds, and low self-concepts in order to survive. That survival was discussed in previous chapters.

TOWARD A NEW IDENTITY

Many persons without disabilities do not understand the seemingly unmitigated rejection they receive from persons with disabilities. While not limited to people with physical disabilities, much of this rejection is given by them. At first glance, it often appears that they are looking for an unprovoked fight. Upon closer examination, their anger is based on a series of rebuffs. A prominent question debated by people with disabilities is, "Should they opt out of peer group relationships with people who do not have disabilities?" In the vernacular of separatist philosophy, should they "think 'disabled,'" "buy 'disabled,'" and otherwise "live as 'disabled people?'" Mindful of the negative implications, it is worthwhile to go beyond emotionalism in order to review some of the sociopsychological conditions that may lead to separatism.

Numerous theorists have stated that the self is both the *subject* and *object* of social interactions. The self is a doer when an individual is actively perceiving, thinking, and remembering things. It is an object when an individual forms his or her attitudes, feelings, and evaluations. Specifically, people with disabilities are not merely recipients of the whims of others; they also make things happen. The view that past and current problems centering on disabilities are problems only of people with disabilities is a grossly oversimplified and inaccurate perception. Such a definition of the situation is analogous to blaming the victim.

The writings of numerous theorists state that all people, regardless of their physical abilities, seek psychological unity, equilibrium, and stability. Alfred Adler (1935) coined the term *creative self* in an effort to describe each individual's unique processes of interpreting his or her life experiences and adjusting his or her behavior in order to achieve psychological balance. There is no single way persons with disabilities respond to psychological disequilibrium: Some individuals become hostile; others clown; still others assume proud mannerisms; many withdraw. The type of adjustment depends to a great extent on learned sociocultural coping mechanisms. Evaluating individual cases, one could argue convincingly that the images individuals have of themselves may be inappropriate for their survival. The self-concepts of persons with disabilities frequently are distorted by adverse environmental conditions, causing them to project an unreasonably low estimate of their self-worth.

A negative self-concept usually results from prolonged conditions of assault on the ego. Just as ethnic minorities' self-concepts are contaminated by a color-caste complex, continued conditions of second-class citizenship dull the aspirations of people with disabilities. For the oppressed minorities and persons with disabilities who try to overcome social and physical barriers, history is replete with illustrations of failures. For example, when researchers examine classrooms occupied by children with disabilities, they are likely to conclude that failure, not success, is the norm. When compiled as a collection of individual experiences, it is a fair estimate that as a whole, persons with disabilities, have a tradition of frustration and failure.

Somewhat similar to Jews in the Nazi concentration camps, individuals with disabilities react to oppression in a wide variety of ways: (1) resignation and defeat, (2) heightened in-group feelings, (3) adoption of temporary frames of security, (4) shifts in levels of aspiration, (5) regression and fantasy, (6) conformity to nondisabled group norms and expectations, (7) changes in philosophy of life, (8) direct action, and (9) aggression and displaced aggression. Of these reactions, resignation and defeat, regression and fantasy, conformity to nondisabled group norms and expectations, and aggression are the behaviors most likely to be expressed in negative self-concepts. Clearly, no single set of environmental conditions automatically causes people with disabilities to adopt negative self-concepts. Most lower-class persons do, however, seem to be insulated against positive self-concepts as a result of their inability to achieve rewards comparable to those of their nondisabled peers. The nebulous white middle class is the positive reference group for most people with disabilities. From early childhood, they, similar to ethnic minorities, are taught to admire or at least achieve white middle-class goals. Once they buy into this system, all other societal norms become secondary. Upwardly aspiring, their dilemma is evident: They cannot choose both the dominant culture and a subculture of disability without experiencing role conflict. Consequently, many persons with disabilities are suspended between the two groups, and their dual membership is a hindrance to their rehabilitation and social integration. Thus, they frequently are torn between asserting their membership either in disabled citizens' groups or in nondisabled citizens' groups, maintaining a schizophrenic identity in both, or denying the attraction of either.

Rejection by people without disabilities has caused many persons with disabilities to abandon the American dream of equality and substitute a new dream, separatism. Again, the authors caution the reader not to attribute a single cause to individuals' joining disability-oriented groups. The real point to be emphasized is that both organized and spontaneous social movements result not because all individuals participating in these movements are identically (and sociologically) motivated but because they have a variety of authentically subjective motives that drive them to seek and find outlets in the same types of collective activity.

To low-achieving individuals, disability-oriented organizations and activities may be viewed as an escape from competition with people who do not have disabilities. To aspiring leaders, these groups may be viewed as a way to offset the effect of competing with able-bodied leaders. To unemployed people with disabilities, these organizations may be seen as an opportunity to get jobs. In short, disability-oriented organizations attract many people who have different needs.

Generally, disability-oriented groups take lower– and middle-class disabled people out of the social arenas that feature nondisabled role models for emulation. At first glance, one might surmise that the displacement of role models who do not have disabilities is a negative adjustment. However, *it is negative only when acceptance by people with disabilities has a strong value*. Otherwise, the valuation of role models with physical disabilities is both bearable and desirable. For people who feel that they can never achieve maximum success in the larger society, these organizations offer norms and activities centering on disabilities and a new hope. Extremists believe that "crips" and "gimps" are lost in ignorance and must seek out their true identity, must gain control over their own economic fortunes by setting up their own living environments and businesses. This position does not have widespread support.

Like the positive effects of psychotherapy, disability-oriented groups have therapeutic value in the strict sense of removing symptoms of inferiority. For example, the therapy results from changing individuals' views of themselves in a positive direction ("Disabled is beautiful.") and altering their view of people who do not have disabilities and their relation to them ("All people are equal."). When based on a rigid code of conduct (such as following approved rehabilitation programs, exhibiting well-mannered behavior, and abstaining from making negative comments about other people), disability-oriented organizations contribute to an orderly society. However, when based on ethnocentrism ("Disabled people are better.") and hatred, these organizations, like their able-bodied counterparts, are socially destructive. Contrary to popular opinion, societal destruction is not the reason most people with disabilities join organizations.

Further, as in any group process, de-individualization, a reduction of inner restraints in individual members, makes possible the negative potential of any organization. Each year that their full citizenship is denied, Americans with disabilities in increasing numbers agree with the assertion that people without disabilities cannot, in general, be taken as models of how to live. Rather, they are themselves in great need of new standards that will release them from their inhumanity and place them once again in contact with the depths of their own humane selves.

Disability-oriented organizations mainly are searching for *disabilitude*, a term the authors use to designate positive self-identity. Oppressive persons have forced individuals with disabilities to ask themselves, "Who am I?" Gradually, the shame of a once-scorned, barbaric, degrading history is giving way to recognizing the many fine contributions made by all individuals. In America this has become a literary and social action movement. Thus, disabilitude is the antithesis of the systematic negation of the disability experience. It is shaped, first, in the lives and writings of persons with disabilities and, second, in local, state, and national activities on behalf of them. Like the phoenix, people with disabilities are rising in a new positive image out of the ashes of the old negative stereotypes.

PROBLEMS OF HELPERS

Successfully helping clients with disabilities does not require gimmicks or tricks. Furthermore, effective helpers use different techniques. There is not just one right approach and many wrong approaches. Indifference or condescension, for example, is an ineffective way to help, while concern and respect have proven to be better. Many clients have been both disappointed and psychologically emasculated by professional and paraprofessional helpers. When this happens, the clients quickly learn to consider a helper guilty of disliking them until he or she proves otherwise. However, once most clients accept a helper, it is almost impossible for the helper to do anything wrong in their eyes.

For the remainder of this section, the authors will discuss social agency-client interactions. Although this is done to narrow the focus of the discussion, the comments are relevant to other situations also.

Generally, low achievement by persons with disabilities is encouraged by the low expectations held by helpers. In most instances, this attitude is fostered by the conscious or unconscious belief in the notion of the physiological and intellectual inferiority of all people with disabilities. Such an attitude can be completely destructive to the education and rehabilitation processes. If individuals with disabilities do poorly in a task, some helpers tend erroneously to perceive the cause of the performance as internal to the clients and thus attribute negative characteristics to them. However, if the clients do well, these helpers take the credit for having overcome formidable odds in order to help the dullards.

It is behavior, not physical difference, that is the crucial quality of rehabilitation. As stated several times, helpers should treat all clients fairly. Hostile clients frequently are provoked to aggressive acts by hostile helpers. The initial error committed by professional helpers is usually to assume that persons with disabilities and those without them are biologically and psychologically different. Each client wants to be treated with respect. Through their behavior, helpers demonstrate the extent of their recognition that each client has worth and dignity. In spite of how difficult it may be to assist some persons with disabilities, helpers must view these persons as individuals who deserve the same opportunity to succeed as those who are believed to be easier to reach. Besides, there is a way to help every client effectively, and each helper must find it.

Clients with disabilities who have been treated with respect and dignity are likely to reciprocate with similar behavior. Most people learn best by example. Children who hate have been conditioned by adults who hate them, while those who love have been the recipients of love. In Chapter 9 the authors noted how important it is that teachers consciously seek to minimize unfair treatment and maximize fair treatment. Showing favoritism to some students and constantly punishing others is enough to suggest to class members that the teacher is more attracted to some students than to others. When students see a teacher rejecting students with disabilities, they may imagine that in order to be liked by the teacher they must reject those students, too. There is nothing creative or imaginative about most forms of rejection. They are merely old-fashioned ways of hatred.

If they wish to be successful working with their clients, helpers must convey the fact that they are concerned with and interested in each of them. Clearly, this should have nothing to do with physiological attributes. It is a matter of equity and professionalism. Helpers who maintain an attitude of fairness to all clients and whose behavior demonstrates it will find their clients with disabilities most receptive to them as helpers and, perhaps, friends. All clients want desperately to be assisted by helpers who care about them.

In many instances, helpers will discover that they must first build confidence in their clients. Believing that clients with disabilities are capable of learning and succeeding is not sufficient.

The clients also must believe it. There are many ways helpers can assist in raising clients' levels of aspiration. It would be cruel to raise them above the point of their realization, but, then, who except persons who really know the clients' condition should make such a crucial determination? Commenting on levels of aspiration of school children, William Wattenberg (1959) wrote:

> The ideal situation for normal children is for their level of aspiration to be just high enough so that they have to put forth effort to reach it, and yet for them to achieve success. In school, at least in the beginning for any subject, children tend to accept the teachers' expectations and standards as their level of aspiration. Therefore, we can influence this level quite effectively. Now, when the level favors success with effort, a number of fine things happen.
>
> The situation itself is satisfying. The child will want to return to the type of task. So to speak, now he is motivated, shows interest, and puts out effort. Moreover, unless he is emotionally disturbed, he will begin to raise his sights. He will set himself after each success a somewhat higher level of aspiration. . . .
>
> If the task at hand is clearly beyond his ability, he fails. What does failure do? Not only does it rob the task of interest, but it can have a depressant effect on his future level of aspiration. His ambitions for himself will curve sharply downward. . . . He sets himself a level considerably below his true ability. [P. 231]

Thus, levels of aspiration are similar to an automobile governor: on the one hand, protecting the disabled against demoralizing failures and, on the other hand, allowing them to experience safe, morale-building successes. Also like a governor, when the mechanism of levels of aspiration is thrown out of balance, it fails to perform its protective function. Under this condition, aspirations may be maintained consistently above or below achievement.

All helpers should remember that behavioral science theories are simply symbolic constructs that allow one to partially account for and to predict human behavior. When studied in this relation, each theory has some potential for adding to knowledge of human behavior. The importance of helpers' not forgetting or repressing this fact is exemplified in the condition of a recent college graduate who, armed with many theories of disabilities, was very much confused by the behavior of the clients who came to him for help. The young man did not realize that most of his clients had not read the theories and, therefore, could not respond as they "should have." His primary task was not to acquaint them with the relevant theories and thereby cause them to behave correctly but instead to expand his theories to include their behavior.

MARGINAL PEOPLE

In many ways, people with disabilities are marginal people. Robert Park (1937) defined a *marginal person* as one whom fate has condemned to live in two societies and in two not merely different but antagonistic cultures. *Marginality* is characterized by the following conditions: (1) There must be a situation that places two cultures or subcultures in lasting contact. In this case, one subculture consists of people with disabilities and another consists of those without disabilities. (2) One culture must be dominant in terms of power and reward potential. Continuing the above illustration, the nondisabled group is dominant. This is the nonmarginal of the two cultures, and its members are not particularly influenced or attracted by groups or organizations of people with disabilities. (3) The boundaries between the two cultures must be sufficiently defined for the members of the marginal (disability) culture to internalize feelings of inferiority and to be unhappy with them.

It is important to acknowledge that not all persons with disabilities are marginal. On the contrary, many of them are well adjusted. However, most persons with disabilities are marginal in reference to other persons, and their marginality is compounded by making them marginal to their socioeconomic peers. Finally, some of them are marginal to other persons with disabilities, e.g. females are marginal to males. When all of these facts coalesce, an accurate picture of people with disabilities is formed. They exhibit marginal characteristics, and many of them have become victims of aspirations that they cannot achieve and hopes that they cannot satisfy.

While most people with disabilities probably aspire to high levels of education and occupations, without considerable assistance and reinforcement, few of them actually expect to achieve such goals. Youths with disabilities, for example, unlike youths without disabilities, tend to expect failure in school tasks. They have seen too many other persons with disabilities who aspired high but achieved low. Besides, seldom are other things equal when persons with disabilities and those who do not have them are compared. Certainly their physical and environmental conditions are not equal: Man has yet to achieve a barrier-free society. Giving individuals opportunities to perform societal tasks does not mean that they will automatically take advantage of the opportunities. This is certainly true in some jobs and academic settings, in which individuals with disabilities seem to require a longer period of adjustment. This delay is related more to various nonremediated barriers than to their abilities.

People with disabilities and people without disabilities usually live in psychological environments that represent microcosmic views of two contrasting and often antagonistic worlds. More imposing is the feeling that they represent alien cultures, neither of which is able to communicate successfully with the other. As a result, they frequently harbor untold fears of each other. Each considers the other to be heartless and somewhat barbaric. When helpers are misinformed about the psyche of their clients, they pass their ignorance on to their clients. Individuals with disabilities too often believe themselves to be inferior to the so-called able-bodied, and the able-bodied too often believe themselves to be superior to them. As a continuing condition, this is a social tragedy in which all the players lose. Unless the cultural restrictions are ameliorated, civil rights laws and regulations will be Shakespearean in nature: full of sound and fury but signifying nothing.

Of the many conclusions that can be drawn from the studies reviewed in this book, it seems worthwhile to note that once people with disabilities perceive that they are able to interact with other people and not be penalized, differences in their aspirations and achievements no longer reflect stereotypes. It is not a single set of conditions that places people with disabilities at a disadvantage when competing with other people. Some of the many conditions include negative parental influence, alienated peers, and nonresponsive professional and paraprofessional helpers.

The authors have spent a large amount of time considering

ways to assist people with disabilities to conform to societal molds, but, they ask, "What is so good about conforming to the standards of the larger society?" In trying to provide, to individuals with disabilities, opportunities to fit into the "normal" world, helpers often ignore the many positive characteristics that are accentuated in the survival of people with disabilities: compassion for less fortunate people, the tendency to see more than physical qualities in other people, and humility during task performance. Of course, one could argue that societal success is measured mainly by standards set by people who do not have disabilities and that therefore this is the best game of survival.

If social consensus defines the shift from a "disabled" category to a "nondisabled" category as being best, does this not rule out the probability of people with permanent disabilities ever feeling totally comfortable, psychologically and socially? Stated another way, does the "good life" by societal definition require no permanent disabilities? Apparently this is the belief of most people. People with disabilities have the statistically least probable chance of achieving educational and occupational success. Does this mean that they also have the statistically least probable chance of being happy? If they accept these standards and values, the answer is yes. A growing number of persons and groups are challenging this myopic view of societal goals and social outcomes, however.

SUMMARY: LESSONS LEARNED FROM HELEN KELLER

There are several famous persons with disabilities whose lives chronicle the triumph of mind over matter (*see* Appendix A). Succinctly, the major lessons to be learned from them are that neither do people think with their eyes and ears and limbs, nor is the capacity for thought determined by the five senses. Helen Keller epitomizes these lessons. Born blind and deaf, she was able to reach within herself to learn from individuals who saw with their eyes, heard with their ears, and spoke with their mouths. However, she did not accomplish this feat alone. With the assistance and patience of Anne Sullivan, her teacher and friend, Helen Keller learned to read and write in Braille before she was ten years old and to speak well enough at age sixteen to go to preparatory school. Later, she attended Radcliffe College, where she graduated with honors in 1904.

In *The Story of My Life,* Ms. Keller (1905) recounted the mental awakening she got from Plato's concept of an "Absolute" that gives inner beauty to the beautiful, music to the musical, and truth to what is called *true* irrespective of one's physical wholeness or disabilities. She found the essence of humanity in Descartes's maxim, "I think, therefore, I am." From this perspective, life is a thinking existence, not the physical shell one occupies during life. Finally, from Kant's writings, Ms. Keller learned that sensations without concepts are barren and concepts without sensations are empty. Drawing on her mind's power, she used thought, smell, and feelings to extrapolate the meanings of things people see and hear.

The human rights laws and advancements of people with disabilities did not begin with Helen Keller, but they certainly were dramatized by her. Teaching speech to the deaf and teaching the use of Braille to the blind in the nineteenth century are two of the greatest advances in the treatment of the physically disabled. Even so, it is still difficult for most people who do not have a disability to understand what it is like to have one. Karl Menninger (1930) explained this insensitivity in words that even nonprofessionals can understand: "When a trout rising to a fly gets hooked on a line and finds himself unable to swim about freely, he begins with a fight which results in struggles and splashes and sometimes an escape. Often, of course, the situation is too tough for him. Sometimes he masters his difficulties; sometimes they are too much for him. His struggles are all that the world sees and it naturally misunderstands them. It is hard for a free fish to understand what is happening to a hooked one" (p. 3).

The deaf who do not speak are isolated from people who hear and talk, for example, and this isolation often is cruelly complete. It is an inhuman silence that severs and estranges the deaf from the nondeaf, not to be broken by words of greeting, songs of birds, or sounds of a breeze. In the United States, a few concerned individuals, like Alexander Graham Bell, did more than talk about deafness. Bell founded and financed the American Association to Promote the Teaching of Speech to the Deaf, in 1890. With the help of this organization, the deaf were brought into the mainstream. So, too, were the blind, with Louis Braille's efforts. As a fifteen-year-old blind French student in the National Institute for the Blind in Paris, Braille developed a raised dot-dash reading system in 1824. In 1829 he published the Braille system, which allowed the blind to read and write. The medical profession had known since 1881 that at least two-thirds of all blindness in children occurred at birth and that the disease that caused this blindness was associated with venereal disease, although not always caused by it. By 1900 a large number of physicians had begun prenatal care to prevent blindness, and, at their urging, lay committees for the prevention of blindness were established.

All of this occurred during Helen Keller's childhood, and she benefited from the advanced methods of treating the blind and the deaf. Were she alive today, she probably would be disappointed at how little national attitudes have changed. Many people still believe that the blind can tell colors by touch and that all blind people are sensitive, shy persons. There is still a tendency also for people to believe that physical disability means inability to be an integral member of the family, school, and community.

This nation has yet to learn from Ms. Keller's life that physical disability should not deprive people of their individuality. Even Ms. Keller forgot this early in her adult life. She believed that because she had overcome deafness and blindness sufficiently to be happy, anyone could do the same if he or she really tried. She forgot that her success was due in part to her family's wealth and in part to helpful persons. She was like a princess in a fairy tale who lived in a palace composed of mirrors that reflected only her image. Belatedly, she learned that the power to overcome a physical disability is not awakened in everyone. Adequate income, top quality education, and friends are but a few of the ingredients for successful rehabilitation. Also, the will to succeed is important.

Survival places the same demands on people with disabilities as those without disabilities and requires the same sacrifices of them; therefore, society should provide all people with the same individual rights. When discussing the rights of people with disabilities, the authors have focused, first, on what they are entitled to as persons; second, on what they have as citizens; and third, on what they need as persons with disabilities. With or without equality, they will play a myriad of social roles. Obviously, they will be better citizens if they are adequately educated, fairly employed, safely housed, and humanely accepted. It is the right of every citizen to receive education for the full development of his or her mind and body and to be completely emancipated from all forms of bondage, superstition, and crippling fear.

No matter how much people with disabilities prefer to be protected and supported by professional helpers or how much helpers desire to protect and support them, clients ultimately are masters of their own lives. Accordingly, each master must be the captain and engineer during his or her journey through life. In nautical terms, this means plotting a course, gauging the social climate, and knowing when and in what direction to travel. Parents, friends, and other helpers are crew members who can relieve the captain of many chores needed to successfully reach the destination, but it is neither their disability nor their life.

Each person comes into this world alone under circumstances unlike those of any other person. True, there are similarities in birth, but each birth is a unique happening. When any person dies, he or she leaves this world alone under circumstances peculiar to himself or herself. The time spent between birth and death also is a unique experience. There can never be a similar combination of nurture and nature. Therefore, all people are unique beings who share common human needs and social systems. When the artificial discriminators are removed and people with disabilities are recognized as individuals, then they are judged and treated on merit.

People with disabilities have proven that they can equal other persons in thought, art, science, literature, and other cultural achievements. Helen Keller's success has been replicated and exceeded by other persons. Individuals with disabilities fill professors' chairs and editors' desks, plead cases at the bar of justice, perform complex medical operations, speak from pulpits, and build them too. Yet, these are mere facades. Helen Keller wanted people to look at the inner selves of persons with disabilities. These inner selves are more hidden than the caves of the gnomes, but once one locates them, one finds human beings.

An old slave poem captures the essence of conditions for people with disabilities:

> We ain't what we ought to be.
> We ain't what we gonna be.
> We ain't what we wanta be.
> But, thank God,
> We ain't what we was.

NOTE TO HELPERS

Helpers should—

1. be kind to themselves!
2. remind themselves that they are helpers, not magicians. They cannot change anyone else. They can only change how they relate to other people.
3. find a quiet place and use it as much as possible to have time with themselves.
4. give encouragement to clients but do not offer them false hope.
5. remember that there will be times when they will feel frustrated, helpless, and inadequate. They should admit these feelings without shame. They are human. Caring and being available to clients may be all that helpers can give at times.
6. learn to recognize the difference between complaining about a job that relieves stress and complaining that reinforces stress.
7. be creative. They should try new approaches to helping clients. However, they should use new approaches only after they understand the implications and feel comfortable with them.
8. use colleagues as a support system. No one has all the answers. Helpers should use their colleagues for consultation and support.
9. say "I choose" rather than "I should," "I have to," "I ought to," say "I won't" rather than "I can't."
10. not apologize for saying no. If they never say no, what is their yes worth?
11. not forget to laugh and play.

REFERENCES

Adler, Alfred. The fundamental views of individual psychology. *J Ind Psychol, 1:* 5–8, 1935.

Keller, Helen. *The Story of My Life.* New York: Doubleday, 1905.

Menninger, Karl. *The Human Mind.* New York: Alfred A. Knopf, 1930.

Park, Robert E. In Stonequist, Everett V. *The Marginal Man.* New York: Charles Scribner's Sons, 1937.

Wattenberg, William W. Levels of aspiration. *MI Educ J, 37:* 231–40, 1959.

Additional Readings

Berger, Clyde C. *Grandpa's Boy and What Became of Him.* Wichita, KS: Rand, 1981.

Brack, Joyce, and Collins, Robert. *One Thing for Tomorrow: A Woman's Personal Struggle with MS.* Saskatchewan, Canada: Western Producer Prairie Books, 1981.

Eisenberg, Myron B., Griggins, Cynthia, and Duval, Richard J. (Eds.). *Disabled People as Second-Class Citizens.* New York: Springer, 1982.

Goldberg, Richard T. *The Making of Franklin D. Roosevelt: Triumph Over Disability.* Cambridge, MA: Abt Books, 1981.

Grief, Elaine, and Matarazzo, Ruth G. *Behavioral Approaches to Rehabilitation.* New York: Springer, 1982.

Nolan, Christopher. *Dam-Burst of Dreams.* Athens: Ohio University Press, 1981.

Zola, Irving K. *Missing Pieces: A Chronicle of Living with a Disability.* Philadelphia: Temple University Press, 1982.

FAMOUS DECEASED PERSONS
WITH DISABILITIES: A BRIEF SAMPLE

A

CLINTON P. ANDERSON (1895–1975) served as Secretary of Agriculture and later as a United States Senator from New Mexico. He had diabetes.

SUSAN B. ANTHONY (1820–1906) was a leading advocate for women's rights and is the first woman honored on a United States coin. She had arthritis.

ARISTOTLE (384–322 BC) was one of the world's greatest philosophers and teachers. He stuttered.

THOMAS R. ARMITAGE (1795–1842), a physician, introduced Braille into England and also spearheaded legislation that mandated compulsory education for the blind between the ages of five and sixteen years. He was partially sighted.

B

BERNARD M. BARUCH (1870–1965) was a successful businessman, elder statesman, and presidential adviser. He was hard-of-hearing.

THOMAS A BECKET (1117–1170) was a member of the clergy who became Archbishop of Canterbury and, after his death, a saint. He stuttered.

JOACHIM DU BELLAY (1522–1560) was a talented poet. He was partially deaf.

LOUIS BRAILLE (1800–1852) invented the Braille system by which blind people can read and write through a planned series of raised dots. He was blind.

ELIZABETH BARRETT BROWNING (1806–1861) was a world-renowned poetess. She had a spinal injury.

RALPH BUNCHE (1904–1971), a physician, served as under secretary general of the United Nations and in 1950 won the Nobel peace prize. He had diabetes.

C

JULIUS CAESAR (100–44 BC) was one of the world's greatest military leaders and a Roman emperor. He had epilepsy.

GEORGE WASHINGTON CARVER (1864–1943) was an outstanding scientist and educator. He is best known for developing hundreds of uses for the peanut. He stuttered.

IRENE CHAVARRIA (1941–1974) was an instructor at East Los Angeles College. She was a quadriplegic.

FANNY CROSBY (1820–1915) was a much-acclaimed teacher of the blind at the New York Institute for the Blind. She was blind.

D

WILLIAM O. DOUGLAS (1898–1980) was a successful lawyer who became an Associate Justice of the United States Supreme Court. He had poliomyelitis as a child.

E

THOMAS A. EDISON (1847–1930) was a famous inventor whose inventions included the incandescent electric lamp and the receiver and transmitter for the automatic telegraph. He was deaf.

ST. JOHN ERVINE (1883–1971) was a well-known writer of novels, plays, biographies, and reviews. He had one leg.

LEONARD EULER (1707–1783) was one of the founders of the science of pure mathematics. He was partially sighted.

F

HENRY FAWCETT (1833–1884) was an economist and statesman who became postmaster general of Britain. He was blind.

GUSTAVE FLAUBERT (1821–1880) was a famous French novelist. He had epilepsy.

G

GALILEO GALILEI (1564–1642) was a famous astronomer and physicist who wrote *The Laws of Motion*. He was blind.

CHARLES GOUNOD (1818–1893) was a celebrated composer whose music includes "Ave Maria" and "Faust." He was blind.

FRANCISCO GOYA (1746–1828) was a royal painter to the King of Spain. He was deaf.

EDWIN GRASSE (1884–1954) was a composer, violinist, and organist. He was blind.

H

HANNIBAL (247–183 BC) led his army with its elephants across the Alps in an unsuccessful attempt to defeat the Romans. He was blind in one eye.

FRANCOIS HUBER (1750–1831) gained fame as a naturalist who became an authority on the honeybee. He was blind.

I

ELIZABETH INCHBALD (1753–1821) was an actress and writer in England. She stuttered.

ISAAC II (1155–1204) ruled the Eastern Roman Empire. He was blind.

J

JAMES JOYCE (1881–1941) gained world recognition as a novelist. He was blind.

K

PHILIP KEARNEY (1814–1862) was a much-decorated Civil War general. He had one arm.

RUDYARD KIPLING (1865–1936) was a successful writer who received a Nobel prize for literature in 1907. He was partially sighted.

CASPAR KRUMBHORN (1542–1621) was a director of the Academy of St. Peter's in Rome. He was blind.

L

FRITZ LANG (1890–1976) was a director of motion pictures. He was blind in one eye.

CANADA LEE (1907–1951) was one of the most successful black actors in the United States in the early twentieth century. He was blind in one eye.

MAXIM LITVINOFF (1876–1951) was Russian Ambassador to the United States in 1941. He had diabetes.

HENRY LUCE (1898–1976) founded and published *Fortune, Time,* and other magazines. He stuttered.

M

ANNE SULLIVAN MACY (1887–1936) was a teacher and life companion of Helen Keller. She was blind in one eye.

HERBERT MARSHALL (1890–1966) was a star of radio, theatre, movies, and television. He had one leg.

EDWARD MARSHALL (1856–1937) founded the *Harvard Lampoon* and *Life Magazine.* He was deaf.

HARRIET MARTINEAU (1802–1876) was an English economist and novelist. She was deaf.

JOHN METCALF (1717–1810), a road builder, was one of the first persons to use crushed stone in roads. He was blind.

N

HORATIO NELSON (1758–1805) was a distinguished English admiral. He was blind in one eye and had one arm amputated.

P

LOUIS PASTEUR (1822–1895) verified the germ theory of disease and developed the process of pasteurization. He was a paralytic.

WILEY POST (1900–1935) was a pioneer in aviation. He had one eye.

WILLIAM PRESCOTT (1796–1859), was a famous historian who wrote classic volumes of Spanish-American history. He was blind in one eye and partially sighted in the other.

JOSEPH PULITZER (1847–1911) endowed Columbia University's

School of Journalism, which in turn established the Pulitzer prizes. He was blind.

R

JOSHUA REYNOLDS (1732–1792) was a famous portrait painter. He was hard-of-hearing.

ANNE ELEANOR ROOSEVELT (1884–1962) is considered by many writers to have been America's greatest first lady. She was hard-of-hearing.

FRANKLIN DELANO ROOSEVELT (1882–1945) was the thirty-second president of the United States and the only president elected to four terms. He was crippled by poliomyelitis.

S

EDWARD SCRIPPS (1854–1926) organized a chain of newspapers throughout the United States and endowed the Scripps Institute of Oceanography in San Diego. He was blind.

MAURICE DE LA SIZERANNE (1857–1924) taught blind students and was a founder of a library and a museum that featured the cultural contributions of blind persons. He was blind.

THOMAS SYDENHAM (1624–1689) was the founder of modern clinical medicine. He had gout.

T

NORMAN THOMAS (1884–1968) was an American Socialist leader and candidate for president of the United States six times. He was vision impaired.

W

EDGAR WALLACE (1875–1932) was a prolific novelist, who wrote *Ben Hur.* He was deaf.

FINAL NOTE

This list of abbreviated achievements is not meant to be exhaustive. Rather, it is presented to show various ways individual efforts can overshadow physical disabilities. The authors encourage readers to try to familiarize themselves with the total achievements of the persons on this list and others who are not included. There are thousands of success stories: Fill in some of the missing ones.

Appendix B

RESOURCES FOR PEOPLE WITH DISABILITIES

Alcoholism

National Council on Alcoholism
733 Third Avenue
New York, NY 10017
Phone: 212-986-4433

Amputation

National Amputation Foundation
12–45 150th Street
Whitestone, NY 11347
Phone: 212-767-0596

Arthritis

Arthritis Foundation
475 Riverside Drive
New York, NY 10027
Phone: 212-678-6363

Blindness or Visual Impairment

American Council of the Blind
1211 Connecticut Avenue, N.W.
Suite 506
Washington, DC 20036
Phone: 202-833-1251

American Foundation for the Blind, Inc.
15 W. 16th Street
New York, NY 10011
Phone: 212-924-0420

American Library Association Library Services to the Blind
    and Physically Handicapped
50 E. Huron Street
Chicago, IL 60611
Phone: 312-944-6780

American Printing House for the Blind
1839 Frankfort Avenue
Louisville, KY 40206
Phone: 502-895-2405

Association for Education of the Visually Handicapped
919 Walnut Street
Fourth Floor
Philadelphia, PA 19107
Phone: 215-924-7555

Braille Circulating Library
2700 Stuart Avenue
Richmond, VA 23220
Phone: 804-359-3743

Christian Record Braille Foundation, Inc.
4444 South 52nd Street
Lincoln, NE 68506
Phone: 402-488-0981

Eye-Bank Association of America, Inc.
3195 Maplewood Avenue
Winston-Salem, NC 27103
Phone: 919-768-0719

Guide Dog Foundation for the Blind
109–19 72nd Avenue
Forest Hills, NY 11375
Phone: 212-263-4885

Guiding Eyes for the Blind, Inc.
106 E. 41st Street
New York, NY 10017
Phone: 212-683-5165

Leader Dogs for the Blind
1039 S. Rochester Road
Rochester, MI 48063
Phone: 313-651-9011

National Association for Visually Handicapped
305 E. 24th Street
17-C
New York, NY 10010
Phone: 212-889-3141

National Braille Association
85 Goodwin Avenue
Midland, NJ 07432
Phone: 201-447-1484

National Society for the Prevention of Blindness, Inc.
79 Madison Avenue
New York, NY 10016
Phone: 212-684-3505

New Eyes for the Needy
549 Millburn Avenue
Short Hills, NJ 07078
Phone: 201-376-4903

Cancer

American Cancer Society
777 Third Avenue
New York, NY 10017
Phone: 212-371-2900

Cerebral Palsy

American Academy for Cerebral Palsy
1255 New Hampshire Avenue, N.W.
Washington, DC 20036
Phone: 202-659-8251

Dental Guidance—Council for Cerebral Palsy
122 E. 23rd Street
New York, NY 10010
Phone: 212-441-7300

United Cerebral Palsy Association, Inc.
66 E. 34th Street
New York, NY 10016
Phone: 212-889-6655

Cystic Fibrosis

Cystic Fibrosis
3379 Peachtree Road, N.E.
Atlanta, GA 30326
Phone: 404-262-1100

Deafness and Hearing Impairment

Deafness Research Foundation
366 Madison Avenue
New York, NY 10017
Phone: 212-682-3737

International Association of Parents of the Deaf
814 Thayer Avenue
Silver Springs, MD 20910
Phone: 301-585-5400

Ministry to the Deaf
Lutheran Church–Missouri Synod
Board of Missions
500 N. Broadway
St. Louis, MO 63102
Phone: 314-231-6969

National Association of the Deaf
814 Thayer Avenue
Silver Springs, MD 20910
Phone: 301-587-1788

National Center for Law and the Deaf
Callaudet College

Florida Avenue & Seventh Street, N.E.
Washington, DC 20002
Phone: 202-447-0445

National Hearing Aid Society
20361 Middlebelt Road
Livona, MI 48152
Phone: 383-478-2610

Registry of Interpreters for the Deaf
P.O. Box 1339
Washington, DC 20013
Phone: 202-447-0511

Teletypewriters for the Deaf, Inc.
P.O. Box 28332
Washington, DC 20005
Phone: 202-347-1676

Diabetes

American Diabetes Association
600 Fifth Avenue
New York, NY 10020
Phone: 212-683-7444

Juvenile Diabetes Foundation
23 E. 26th Street
New York, NY 10010
Phone: 212-689-7868

Epilepsy

Epilepsy Foundation of America
1828 L Street, N.W.
Washington, DC 20036
Phone: 202-293-2930

National Epilepsy League
6 N. Michigan Avenue
Chicago, IL 60602
Phone: 312-322-6888

Heart

American Heart Association
7320 Greenville Avenue
Dallas, TX 75231
Phone: 214-750-5414

Hemophilia

National Hemophilia Foundation
25 W. 39th Street
New York, NY 10018
Phone: 212-869-9740

Kidney

National Kidney Foundation
116 E. 27th Street
New York, NY 10016
Phone: 212-889-2210

Lung

American Lung Association
1740 Broadway
New York, NY 10019
Phone: 212-245-8000

Multiple Sclerosis

National Multiple Sclerosis Society
205 E. 42nd Street
New York, NY 10017
Phone: 212-532-3060

Muscular Dystrophy

Muscular Dystrophy Association, Inc.
810 Seventh Avenue
New York, NY 10019
Phone: 212-586-0808

Occupational Therapy

American Occupational Therapy Association
6000 Executive Boulevard
Rockville, MD 20852
Phone: 301-770-2200

Paraplegia

National Paraplegia Foundation
333 N. Michigan Avenue
Chicago, IL 60601
Phone: 312-346-4779

Parkinson's Disease

National Parkinson's Foundation
1501 N.W. Ninth Avenue
Miami, FL 33136
Phone: 305-324-0156

Parkinson's Disease Foundation, Inc.
William Black Medical Research Building
Columbia Presbyterian Medical Center
640 W. 168th Street
New York, NY 10032
Phone: 212-923-4700

American Parkinson's Disease Association, Inc.
147 E. 50th Street
Suite 103
New York, NY 10022
Phone: 212-421-5890

Physical Therapy

American Physical Therapy Association
1156 15th Street, N.W.
Washington, DC 20005
Phone: 202-895-2405

Rehabilitation

National Rehabilitation Counseling Association
1522 K Street, N.W.
Washington, DC 20005
Phone: 202-296-6080

Rehabilitation International U.S.A.
20 W. 40th Street
New York, NY 10018
Phone: 212-869-9907

Sickle Cell Disease

Center for Sickle Cell Disease
2121 Georgia Avenue, N.W.
Washington, DC 20059
Phone: 202-636-7930

Spina Bifida

Spina Bifida Association of America
209 Shiloh Drive
Madison, WI 53705
Phone: 608-836-8969

Other Resources

American Coalition of Citizens With Disabilities
1224 Dupont Circle Blvd.
Room 308
Washington, DC 20036
Phone: 202-785-4265

Boy Scouts of America for the Handicapped Division
US Route 1 & 130
North Brunswick, NJ 08902
Phone: 201-249-6000

Disabled American Veterans
3725 Alexandria Pike
Cold Springs, KY 41076
Phone: 606-441-7300

Girl Scouts of the U.S.A.
Scouting for Handicapped Girls Program
830 Third Avenue
New York, NY 10022
Phone: 212-751-6900

Goodwill Industries of America, Inc.
9200 Wisconsin Avenue
Washington, DC 20016
Phone: 202-520-6500

National Clearinghouse of Rehabilitation
Training Materials
Oklahoma State University
Stillwater, OK 74074
Phone: 405-624-6030

National Easter Seal Society
2023 W. Ogden Avenue
Chicago, IL 60612
Phone: 312-243-8400

Appendix C

RECREATION ASSOCIATIONS

American Blind Bowling Association
150 N. Bellaire Avenue
Louisville, KY 40206
Phone: 502-896-8039

American Wheelchair Bowling Association
2635 N.W. 19th Street
Pompano Beach, FL 33062
Phone: 305-941-1238

National Inconvenienced Sportsmen's Association
3738 Walnut Avenue
Carmichael, CA 95608
Phone: 916-484-2152

National Wheelchair Athletic Association
40–24 62nd Street
Woodside, NY 11377
Phone: 212-424-2929

National Wheelchair Basketball Association
110 Seaton Center
University of Kentucky
Lexington, KY 40506
Phone: 606-257-1523

North America Riding for the Handicapped Association, Inc.
P.O. Box 100
Ashburn, VA 22011
Phone: 730-777-3540

Travel Information Center
Moss Rehabilitation Hospital
12th Street and Tabor Road
Philadelphia, PA 19141
Phone: 215-329-5715

United States Deaf Skiers Association
2 Sunset Hill Road
Simsbury, CT 06070
Phone: 203-244-3341

DISABILITIES QUIZ

The purpose of this quiz is to see how knowledgeable you are about selected aspects of disabilities. *This is not an intelligence test.* You may be quite intelligent regarding disabilities but score low on this quiz, and vice versa. The purpose of this quiz is to challenge and enlighten you regarding specific information. Nothing short of an extensive battery of tests and observations by experts will adequately measure your sensitivity to people who have disabilities. This quiz does not meet these criteria. When supplemented with other information, this quiz can help you to get in touch with your overall knowledge of disabilities.

The *Disabilities Quiz* is designed to be self-administered and self-scored. The degree of your "disability" is presented to remind you that labeling can be self-debasing. What you learn from the quiz is more important than your initial score. There is nothing wrong with not knowing answers to the questions. However, depending on your needs, there may be something wrong if you continually miss the answers. For optimum effectiveness, complete this quiz before reading the text and again after you finish it.

Allow fifteen minutes to answer the questions. Write your answers on a separate sheet of paper. Write the letter of the response that is the most correct answer for each question.

1. Which word does not belong?
   a. Crips
   b. Retards
   c. Gimps
   d. Splibs
2. This disease is characterized by abnormally thick mucus that forms plugs in body organs.

   a. Muscular dystrophy
   b. Cystic fibrosis
   c. Multiple sclerosis
   d. Cerebral palsy

3. All but which of the following are major conditions of cerebral palsy?
   a. Spastic
   b. Deafness
   c. Ataxia
   d. Rigidity

4. Which is the largest open minority group in the United States?
   a. Black Americans
   b. Females
   c. Hispanic Americans
   d. People with disabilities

5. The stages of grief in the order they generally occur are
   a. Denial, anger, bargaining, depression, acceptance
   b. Anger, denial, depression, bargaining, acceptance
   c. Denial, bargaining, anger, depression, acceptance
   d. Bargaining, anger, denial, depression, acceptance

6. Being blind in one eye did not prevent him from becoming a famous actor:
   a. Art Carney
   b. Peter Falk
   c. George Kennedy
   d. Raymond Burr

7. Which statement is false?
   a. Physical disabilities are more readily accepted than mental ones.
   b. A mentally ill middle-class person is less stigmatized than a mentally ill lower-class person.
   c. The basic needs of most people with disabilities are different than those of most people without disabilities.
   d. Except for the limitations imposed by their impairments, people with disabilities are no different than people without disabilities.

8. The positive reference group for most people with disabilities is
   a. Middle-class people with disabilities

b. Lower-class people with disabilities

c. Middle-class people without disabilities

d. Lower-class people without disabilities

9. The largest group of students with disabilities are
   a. Partially sighted
   b. Speech impaired
   c. Orthopedically disabled
   d. Hard-of-hearing

10. A college graduate with a disability who shifts the responsibility for his alcoholism to nondisabled people is likely to be engaging in which defense mechanism?
    a. Projection
    b. Displacement
    c. Repression
    d. Compensation

11. The primary source of security and support for people with disabilities is
    a. Professional helpers
    b. Peer groups
    c. Employers
    d. The family

12. Which statement is false?
    a. Men with disabilities are more likely to be employed than women with disabilities.
    b. Males with disabilities are more likely to be referred to vocational training than females with disabilities.
    c. There is a larger percentage of female heads of households with disabilities than male heads of households with disabilities.
    d. Women with disabilities are less likely than women without disabilities to get a divorce.

13. This renowned Roman had epilepsy:
    a. Cicero
    b. Appius Claudius
    c. Pontius Lupus
    d. Julius Caesar

14. Which is not a major kind of barrier for most people with physical disabilities?

    a. Intellectual
    b. Housing
    c. Architectural
    d. Recreation

15. Which person does not belong in this list?
    a. Captain Hook
    b. Richard III
    c. Peter Pan
    d. Quasimoto

16. In ancient Rome infants with disabilities were
    a. Worshipped as gods
    b. Killed by their fathers
    c. Drowned in the Ganges River
    d. Considered intellectual geniuses

17. Prior to the Civil War, hospitals for the care of persons with physical disabilities were established in
    a. New York and Philadelphia
    b. Boston and Cleveland
    c. St. Louis and Chicago
    d. Indianapolis and Detroit

18. The Goodwill Industries was organized in the United States in 1902 by this person:
    a. Edgar Helms
    b. Helen Keller
    c. William Booth
    d. Jane Addams

19. The first Board of Vocational Education was founded under this act in 1918:
    a. The Smith-Fess Act
    b. The Barden-LaFollette Act
    c. The Social Security Act
    d. The Smith-Sears Act

20. Partial or complete paralysis of two limbs on the same side of the body is called
    a. Monoplegia
    b. Diplegia
    c. Hemiplegia

    d. Paraplegia
21. Not even speaking with a stutter detracted from the contribution of this person:
    a. Booker T. Washington
    b. W. B. DuBois
    c. Malcolm X
    d. George Washington Carver
22. Physiological causes of deafness include
    a. Bad teeth
    b. Malnutrition
    c. Inflammation of the middle ear
    d. All of the above
    e. None of the above
23. This disease attacks the brain and spinal cord:
    a. Multiple sclerosis
    b. Cystic fibrosis
    c. Osteoarthritis
    d. Cerebral palsy
24. Which of the following are the victims of the most discrimination?
    a. Nonwhite females with disabilities
    b. White males with disabilities
    c. White females with disabilities
    d. Nonwhite males with disabilities
25. The inability of an individual to function adequately in a work setting because of barriers created by internal fears is called
    a. A physical handicap
    b. An emotional disability
    c. A social disability
    d. A physical disability
26. She was the first deaf person to have a lead role on Broadway, and she won a Tony award in 1980 for her performance in *Children of a Lesser God:*
    a. Helen Hayes
    b. Priscilla Rounds
    c. Phyllis Frelich
    d. Patti LuPone

27. Which physical disability does not belong in this list?
    a. Cerebral palsy
    b. Paraplegia
    c. Diabetes mellitus
    d. Spina bifida
28. Most lower-class children with disabilities come from homes characterized as
    a. Lacking substantial material objects but receiving enough warmth and parental support
    b. Lacking substantial material objects and parental support
    c. Having adequate material objects but lacking parental warmth and support
    d. Having adequate material objects and parental warmth
29. Antidisability attitudes tend to be well developed in children first around this age:
    a. Three
    b. Ten
    c. Seventeen
    d. Twenty
30. Public Law 94-142 is also known as the
    a. Vocational Rehabilitation Act
    b. Architectural Barriers Act
    c. Education for All Handicapped Children Act
    d. Veteran's Rehabilitation Act
31. This gifted athlete continued playing baseball after losing a leg in an automobile accident:
    a. Bill Toomey
    b. Jack Pardee
    c. Lou Gehrig
    d. Monty Stratton
32. Which is likely to be the most dominant factor in the life of a middle-class black woman with a disability?
    a. Her ethnic identity
    b. Her disability
    c. Her social class
    d. Her sex
33. Which of the following is the single most difficult aspect of nonverbal communication when helpers are dealing with clients who have disabilities?

a. Eye contact
b. Manner of speaking
c. Touching
d. Smiling

34. Title V, Section 504, of the Rehabilitation Act of 1973 provides for
    a. Barrier-free federal buildings
    b. Nondiscrimination of the physically disabled in all federally funded programs
    c. Establishment of an Interagency Committee on Handicapped Employees
    d. None of these

35. Attitudes about people with disabilities are
    a. Seldom formed by logic
    b. Formed as a function of intelligence
    c. Usually formed by personal experience
    d. None of the above

36. Which of the following is true?
    a. People with disabilities are not seen by high status people as social and economic threats.
    b. People with disabilities are a distinct cultural group.
    c. People with disabilities are a unique ethnic group.
    d. People with disabilities become handicapped in a way that parallels racial and ethnic characteristics.

37. Most American Indians with disabilities can be found
    a. On reservations
    b. In the inner cities
    c. In the suburbs
    d. In small towns

38. Federal law requires that job applicants with disabilities
    a. Fill out separate employment forms
    b. Take the same tests as applicants without disabilities
    c. Be given a different interview than applicants without disabilities
    d. Be hired if the company has not filled its quota of workers with disabilities

39. This famous actress has diabetes:
    a. Mary Tyler Moore
    b. Meryl Streep

    c. Liza Minnelli

    d. Sally Field

40. This United States Senator from Hawaii lost his right arm in Italy as a soldier during World War II:

    a. Cooper Brown

    b. Spark Matsunaga

    c. Daniel Inouye

    d. Daniel Akaka

41. This famous composer was blind. Two of his compositions were "Ave Maria" and "Faust":

    a. Franz Schubert

    b. Charles Gounod

    c. George Handel

    d. Peter Tchaikovsky

42. This is a major cause of orthopedic disabilities:

    a. Rheumatic fever

    b. Brain injury

    c. Infantile paralysis

    d. All of the above

    e. None of the above

43. Which is the most crucial factor in determining whether persons with disabilities will make satisfactory adjustment to their disability?

    a. Skilled rehabilitation counselors

    b. Their families

    c. Attitudes of society

    d. Extent of the disabilities

44. Which of the following is normal behavior for parents of children with disabilities?

    a. To want to protect them from emotional hurt

    b. To feel guilty and ashamed

    c. To grieve

    d. All of the above

    e. None of the above

45. This outstanding historian suffered from gout:

    a. Edward Gibbon

    b. Allan Nevin

    c. Edward Channing

    e. William Prescott
46. His deafness was overshadowed by his painting ability:
    a. El Greco
    b. Van Gogh
    c. Goya
    d. Rembrandt
47. Which of the following statements is true?
    a. Men are more likely to have diabetes than women.
    b. Middle-class people are more likely to have diabetes than lower-class people.
    c. Whites are more likely to have diabetes than nonwhites.
    d. All of the above are true.
    e. None of the above is true.
48. Within American ethnic minority families, persons with physical disabilities generally are
    a. Treated like cripples
    b. Loved as persons
    c. Considered bad omens
    d. Not wanted
49. Which of the following statements is true?
    a. Workers with disabilities are likely to injure themselves.
    b. Insurance companies will not let employers hire workers with disabilities.
    c. As a group, workers with disabilities are absent from their jobs more than workers without disabilities.
    d. All of the above are true.
    e. None of the above is true.
50. Ray Charles is to music what Henry Luce is to
    a. Journalism
    b. Law
    c. Mathematics
    d. Theatre

ANSWERS

1. d	11. d	21. d	31. d	41. b
2. b	12. d	22. d	32. b	42. d
3. b	13. d	23. a	33. c	43. b
4. d	14. a	24. a	34. b	44. d
5. a	15. c	25. b	35. a	45. a
6. b	16. b	26. c	36. a	46. c
7. c	17. a	27. c	37. a	47. e
8. c	18. a	28. a	38. b	48. b
9. b	19. d	29. b	39. a	49. e
10. a	20. c	30. c	40. c	50. a

SCORE

45–50	No disability in terms of this quiz
40–44	Slight disability
35–39	Moderate disability
30–34	Severe disability
Less than 30	Profound disability

A word of caution: Your disability, if any, will become a handicap if the information you do not know adversely affects your interactions with persons with disabilities.

NAME INDEX

SUBJECT INDEX